Food Diary

&

Blood Sugar Log

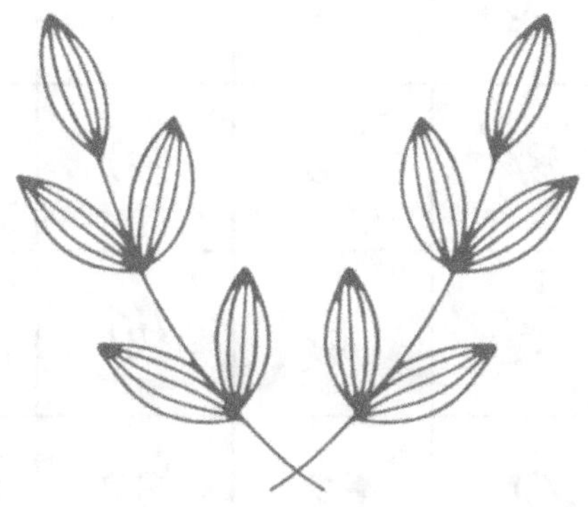

This Book Belongs To

WORKOUT CALENDAR

WEEK 1	1	2	3	4	5	6	7
WEEK 2	8	9	10	11	12	13	14
WEEK 3	15	16	17	18	19	20	21
WEEK 4	22	23	24	25	26	27	28
WEEK 5	29	30	31	32	33	34	35
WEEK 6	36	37	38	39	40	41	42
WEEK 7	43	44	45	46	47	48	49
WEEK 8	50	51	52	53	54	55	56
WEEK 9	57	58	59	60	61	62	63
WEEK 10	64	65	66	67	68	69	70
WEEK 11	71	72	73	74	75	76	77
WEEK 12	78	79	80	81	82	83	84
WEEK 13	85	86	87	88	89	90	

My Goals

- -

- -

- -

- -

Body Measurements/Sizing	
Weight (pounds)	
Waist (inches)	
Chest (inches)	
Hips (inches)	
Estimated Lean Body Weight	
Body Fat Weight Estimated	
Body Fat Percentage Estimated Body Mass Index (BMI)	

Date______/______/______   Day:________   MO TU WE TH FR SA SU

Daily Food and Beverage Log

Food	BREAKFAST				
	Cals	Carbs	Fiber	Protein	Sugar
MEAL SUBTOTAL					

Food	LUNCH				
	Cals	Carbs	Fiber	Protein	Sugar
MEAL SUBTOTAL					

Food	DINNER				
	Cals	Carbs	Fiber	Protein	Sugar
MEAL SUBTOTAL					

Food	SNACKS				
	Cals	Carbs	Fiber	Protein	Sugar
MEAL SUBTOTAL					

DAILY GRAND TOTAL	Cals	Carbs	Fiber	Protein	Sugar	Met my goals today?	Yes	No

WORKOUT LOG

The exercise program and provides.

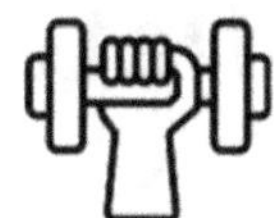

WEIGHT:	
SLEEP (hrs):	
CALORIES:	
TIME (minutes):	

Vitamin/ Supplements/ Meds

....

....

....

EXERCISES	SETS	Duration	Intensity	Cal/Burn

Blood Sugar Log	Before	After	Insulin
Breakfast			
Lunch			
Dinner			
Bedtime			

Note

____

____

Mood

Date___/___/___   Day: ______   MO TU WE TH FR SA SU

Daily Food and Beverage Log

Food	BREAKFAST				
	Cals	Carbs	Fiber	Protein	Sugar
MEAL SUBTOTAL					

Food	LUNCH				
	Cals	Carbs	Fiber	Protein	Sugar
MEAL SUBTOTAL					

Food	DINNER				
	Cals	Carbs	Fiber	Protein	Sugar
MEAL SUBTOTAL					

Food	SNACKS				
	Cals	Carbs	Fiber	Protein	Sugar
MEAL SUBTOTAL					

DAILY GRAND TOTAL	Cals	Carbs	Fiber	Protein	Sugar	Met my goals today?	Yes	No

WORKOUT LOG

The exercise program and provides.

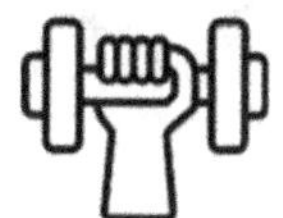

WEIGHT:	
SLEEP (hrs):	
CALORIES:	
TIME (minutes):	

EXERCISES	SETS	Duration	Intensity	Cal/Burn

Blood Sugar Log	Before	After	Insulin
Breakfast			
Lunch			
Dinner			
Bedtime			

Note

Mood

Date___/___/___   Day:______   MO TU WE TH FR SA SU

Daily Food and Beverage Log

Food	BREAKFAST				
	Cals	Carbs	Fiber	Protein	Sugar
MEAL SUBTOTAL					

Food	LUNCH				
	Cals	Carbs	Fiber	Protein	Sugar
MEAL SUBTOTAL					

Food	DINNER				
	Cals	Carbs	Fiber	Protein	Sugar
MEAL SUBTOTAL					

Food	SNACKS				
	Cals	Carbs	Fiber	Protein	Sugar
MEAL SUBTOTAL					

DAILY GRAND TOTAL	Cals	Carbs	Fiber	Protein	Sugar	Met my goals today?	Yes	No

WORKOUT LOG

The exercise program and provides.

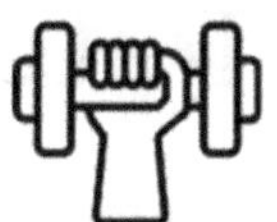

WEIGHT:	
SLEEP (hrs):	
CALORIES:	
TIME (minutes):	

Vitamin / Supplements / Meds

....

....

....

EXERCISES	SETS	Duration	Intensity	Cal/Burn

Blood Sugar Log	Before	After	Insulin
Breakfast			
Lunch			
Dinner			
Bedtime			

Note

____

____

Mood

Date____/____/____   Day:______   MO TU WE TH FR SA SU

Daily Food and Beverage Log

Food	BREAKFAST				
	Cals	Carbs	Fiber	Protein	Sugar
MEAL SUBTOTAL					

Food	LUNCH				
	Cals	Carbs	Fiber	Protein	Sugar
MEAL SUBTOTAL					

Food	DINNER				
	Cals	Carbs	Fiber	Protein	Sugar
MEAL SUBTOTAL					

Food	SNACKS				
	Cals	Carbs	Fiber	Protein	Sugar
MEAL SUBTOTAL					

DAILY GRAND TOTAL	Cals	Carbs	Fiber	Protein	Sugar	Met my goals today?	Yes	No

WORKOUT LOG

The exercise program and provides.

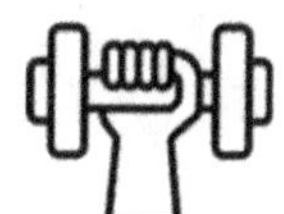

WEIGHT:	
SLEEP (hrs):	
CALORIES:	
TIME (minutes):	

EXERCISES	SETS	Duration	Intensity	Cal/Burn

Blood Sugar Log	Before	After	Insulin
Breakfast			
Lunch			
Dinner			
Bedtime			

Note

Mood

Date ___ / ___ / ___   Day: _______   MO TU WE TH FR SA SU

Daily Food and Beverage Log

Food	BREAKFAST				
	Cals	Carbs	Fiber	Protein	Sugar
MEAL SUBTOTAL					

Food	LUNCH				
	Cals	Carbs	Fiber	Protein	Sugar
MEAL SUBTOTAL					

Food	DINNER				
	Cals	Carbs	Fiber	Protein	Sugar
MEAL SUBTOTAL					

Food	SNACKS				
	Cals	Carbs	Fiber	Protein	Sugar
MEAL SUBTOTAL					

DAILY GRAND TOTAL	Cals	Carbs	Fiber	Protein	Sugar	Met my goals today?	Yes	No

WORKOUT LOG

The exercise program and provides.

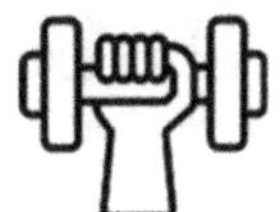

WEIGHT:	
SLEEP (hrs):	
CALORIES:	
TIME (minutes):	

Vitamin/ Supplements/ Meds

....

....

....

EXERCISES	SETS	Duration	Intensity	Cal/Burn

Blood Sugar Log	Before	After	Insulin
Breakfast			
Lunch			
Dinner			
Bedtime			

Note

____

____

Mood

Date____/____/____   Day:______   MO TU WE TH FR SA SU

Daily Food and Beverage Log

Food	BREAKFAST				
	Cals	Carbs	Fiber	Protein	Sugar
MEAL SUBTOTAL					

Food	LUNCH				
	Cals	Carbs	Fiber	Protein	Sugar
MEAL SUBTOTAL					

Food	DINNER				
	Cals	Carbs	Fiber	Protein	Sugar
MEAL SUBTOTAL					

Food	SNACKS				
	Cals	Carbs	Fiber	Protein	Sugar
MEAL SUBTOTAL					

DAILY GRAND TOTAL	Cals	Carbs	Fiber	Protein	Sugar	Met my goals today?	Yes	No

WORKOUT LOG

The exercise program and provides.

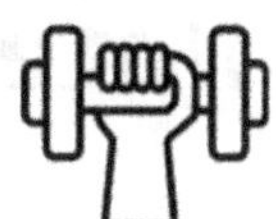

WEIGHT:	
SLEEP (hrs):	
CALORIES:	
TIME (minutes):	

Vitamin/ Supplements/ Meds

....

....

....

EXERCISES	SETS	Duration	Intensity	Cal/Burn

Blood Sugar Log	Before	After	Insulin
Breakfast			
Lunch			
Dinner			
Bedtime			

Note

____

____

Mood

Daily Food and Beverage Log

Date ____ / ____ / ____   Day: ______   MO TU WE TH FR SA SU

Food	BREAKFAST				
	Cals	Carbs	Fiber	Protein	Sugar
MEAL SUBTOTAL					

Food	LUNCH				
	Cals	Carbs	Fiber	Protein	Sugar
MEAL SUBTOTAL					

Food	DINNER				
	Cals	Carbs	Fiber	Protein	Sugar
MEAL SUBTOTAL					

Food	SNACKS				
	Cals	Carbs	Fiber	Protein	Sugar
MEAL SUBTOTAL					

DAILY GRAND TOTAL	Cals	Carbs	Fiber	Protein	Sugar	Met my goals today?	Yes	No

WORKOUT LOG

The exercise program and provides.

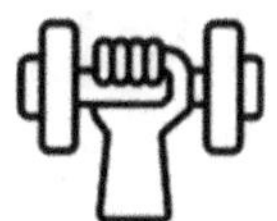

WEIGHT:	
SLEEP (hrs):	
CALORIES:	
TIME (minutes):	

Vitamin/ Supplements/ Meds

....

....

....

EXERCISES	SETS	Duration	Intensity	Cal/Burn

Blood Sugar Log	Before	After	Insulin
Breakfast			
Lunch			
Dinner			
Bedtime			

Note

____

____

Mood

Date_____/_____/_____   Day: _______   MO TU WE TH FR SA SU

Daily Food and Beverage Log

Food	BREAKFAST				
	Cals	Carbs	Fiber	Protein	Sugar
MEAL SUBTOTAL					

Food	LUNCH				
	Cals	Carbs	Fiber	Protein	Sugar
MEAL SUBTOTAL					

Food	DINNER				
	Cals	Carbs	Fiber	Protein	Sugar
MEAL SUBTOTAL					

Food	SNACKS				
	Cals	Carbs	Fiber	Protein	Sugar
MEAL SUBTOTAL					

DAILY GRAND TOTAL	Cals	Carbs	Fiber	Protein	Sugar	Met my goals today?	Yes	No

WORKOUT LOG

The exercise program and provides.

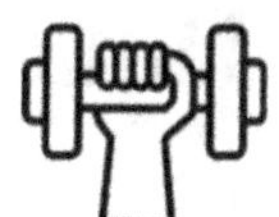

WEIGHT:	
SLEEP (hrs):	
CALORIES:	
TIME (minutes):	

Vitamin/ Supplements/ Meds

....

....

....

EXERCISES	SETS	Duration	Intensity	Cal/Burn

Blood Sugar Log	Before	After	Insulin
Breakfast			
Lunch			
Dinner			
Bedtime			

Note

____

____

Mood

Date____/____/____   Day:______   MO TU WE TH FR SA SU

Daily Food and Beverage Log

Food	BREAKFAST				
	Cals	Carbs	Fiber	Protein	Sugar
MEAL SUBTOTAL					

Food	LUNCH				
	Cals	Carbs	Fiber	Protein	Sugar
MEAL SUBTOTAL					

Food	DINNER				
	Cals	Carbs	Fiber	Protein	Sugar
MEAL SUBTOTAL					

Food	SNACKS				
	Cals	Carbs	Fiber	Protein	Sugar
MEAL SUBTOTAL					

DAILY GRAND TOTAL	Cals	Carbs	Fiber	Protein	Sugar	Met my goals today?	Yes	No

WORKOUT LOG

The exercise program and provides.

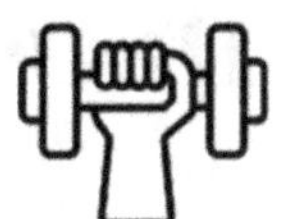

WEIGHT:	
SLEEP (hrs):	
CALORIES:	
TIME (minutes):	

EXERCISES	SETS	Duration	Intensity	Cal/Burn

Blood Sugar Log	Before	After	Insulin
Breakfast			
Lunch			
Dinner			
Bedtime			

Note

Mood

Date____/____/____   Day:______   MO TU WE TH FR SA SU

Daily Food and Beverage Log

Food	BREAKFAST				
	Cals	Carbs	Fiber	Protein	Sugar
MEAL SUBTOTAL					

Food	LUNCH				
	Cals	Carbs	Fiber	Protein	Sugar
MEAL SUBTOTAL					

Food	DINNER				
	Cals	Carbs	Fiber	Protein	Sugar
MEAL SUBTOTAL					

Food	SNACKS				
	Cals	Carbs	Fiber	Protein	Sugar
MEAL SUBTOTAL					

DAILY GRAND TOTAL	Cals	Carbs	Fiber	Protein	Sugar	Met my goals today?	Yes	No

WORKOUT LOG

The exercise program and provides.

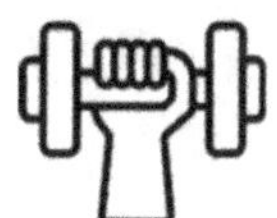

WEIGHT:	
SLEEP (hrs):	
CALORIES:	
TIME (minutes):	

EXERCISES	SETS	Duration	Intensity	Cal/Burn

Blood Sugar Log	Before	After	Insulin
Breakfast			
Lunch			
Dinner			
Bedtime			

Note

Mood

Date____/____/____   Day: ______   MO TU WE TH FR SA SU

Daily Food and Beverage Log

Food	BREAKFAST				
	Cals	Carbs	Fiber	Protein	Sugar
MEAL SUBTOTAL					

Food	LUNCH				
	Cals	Carbs	Fiber	Protein	Sugar
MEAL SUBTOTAL					

Food	DINNER				
	Cals	Carbs	Fiber	Protein	Sugar
MEAL SUBTOTAL					

Food	SNACKS				
	Cals	Carbs	Fiber	Protein	Sugar
MEAL SUBTOTAL					

DAILY GRAND TOTAL	Cals	Carbs	Fiber	Protein	Sugar	Met my goals today?	Yes	No

WORKOUT LOG

The exercise program and provides.

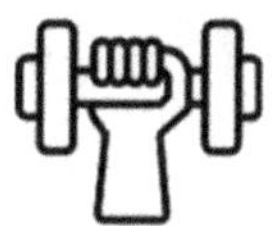

WEIGHT:	
SLEEP (hrs):	
CALORIES:	
TIME (minutes):	

Vitamin/ Supplements/ Meds

....

....

....

EXERCISES	SETS	Duration	Intensity	Cal/Burn

Blood Sugar Log	Before	After	Insulin
Breakfast			
Lunch			
Dinner			
Bedtime			

Note

____

____

Mood

Date___/___/___   Day: ______   MO TU WE TH FR SA SU

Daily Food and Beverage Log

Food	BREAKFAST				
	Cals	Carbs	Fiber	Protein	Sugar
MEAL SUBTOTAL					

Food	LUNCH				
	Cals	Carbs	Fiber	Protein	Sugar
MEAL SUBTOTAL					

Food	DINNER				
	Cals	Carbs	Fiber	Protein	Sugar
MEAL SUBTOTAL					

Food	SNACKS				
	Cals	Carbs	Fiber	Protein	Sugar
MEAL SUBTOTAL					

DAILY GRAND TOTAL	Cals	Carbs	Fiber	Protein	Sugar	Met my goals today?	Yes	No

WORKOUT LOG

The exercise program and provides.

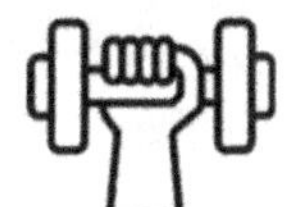

WEIGHT:	
SLEEP (hrs):	
CALORIES:	
TIME (minutes):	

EXERCISES	SETS	Duration	Intensity	Cal/Burn

Blood Sugar Log	Before	After	Insulin
Breakfast			
Lunch			
Dinner			
Bedtime			

Note

Mood

Daily Food and Beverage Log

Date______/______/______   Day: ______   MO TU WE TH FR SA SU

Food	BREAKFAST				
	Cals	Carbs	Fiber	Protein	Sugar
MEAL SUBTOTAL					

Food	LUNCH				
	Cals	Carbs	Fiber	Protein	Sugar
MEAL SUBTOTAL					

Food	DINNER				
	Cals	Carbs	Fiber	Protein	Sugar
MEAL SUBTOTAL					

Food	SNACKS				
	Cals	Carbs	Fiber	Protein	Sugar
MEAL SUBTOTAL					

DAILY GRAND TOTAL	Cals	Carbs	Fiber	Protein	Sugar	Met my goals today?	Yes	No

WORKOUT LOG

The exercise program and provides.

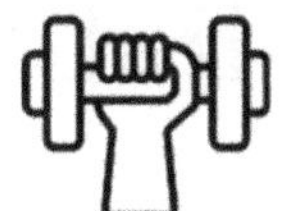

WEIGHT:	
SLEEP (hrs):	
CALORIES:	
TIME (minutes):	

EXERCISES	SETS	Duration	Intensity	Cal/Burn

Blood Sugar Log	Before	After	Insulin
Breakfast			
Lunch			
Dinner			
Bedtime			

Note

Mood

Date___/___/___ Day: ______ MO TU WE TH FR SA SU

Daily Food and Beverage Log

Food	BREAKFAST				
	Cals	Carbs	Fiber	Protein	Sugar
MEAL SUBTOTAL					

Food	LUNCH				
	Cals	Carbs	Fiber	Protein	Sugar
MEAL SUBTOTAL					

Food	DINNER				
	Cals	Carbs	Fiber	Protein	Sugar
MEAL SUBTOTAL					

Food	SNACKS				
	Cals	Carbs	Fiber	Protein	Sugar
MEAL SUBTOTAL					

DAILY GRAND TOTAL	Cals	Carbs	Fiber	Protein	Sugar	Met my goals today?	Yes	No

WORKOUT LOG

The exercise program and provides.

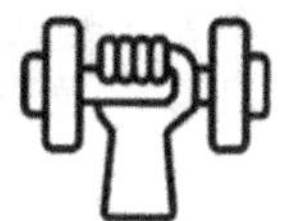

WEIGHT:	
SLEEP (hrs):	
CALORIES:	
TIME (minutes):	

Vitamin / Supplements / Meds

EXERCISES	SETS	Duration	Intensity	Cal/Burn

Blood Sugar Log	Before	After	Insulin
Breakfast			
Lunch			
Dinner			
Bedtime			

Note

Mood

Date___/___/___   Day: ______   MO TU WE TH FR SA SU

Daily Food and Beverage Log

Food	BREAKFAST				
	Cals	Carbs	Fiber	Protein	Sugar
MEAL SUBTOTAL					

Food	LUNCH				
	Cals	Carbs	Fiber	Protein	Sugar
MEAL SUBTOTAL					

Food	DINNER				
	Cals	Carbs	Fiber	Protein	Sugar
MEAL SUBTOTAL					

Food	SNACKS				
	Cals	Carbs	Fiber	Protein	Sugar
MEAL SUBTOTAL					

DAILY GRAND TOTAL	Cals	Carbs	Fiber	Protein	Sugar	Met my goals today?	Yes	No

WORKOUT LOG

The exercise program and provides.

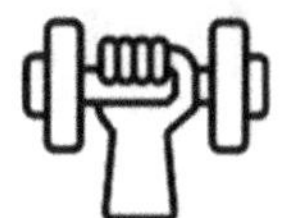

WEIGHT:	
SLEEP (hrs):	
CALORIES:	
TIME (minutes):	

Vitamin/ Supplements/ Meds

....

....

....

EXERCISES	SETS	Duration	Intensity	Cal/Burn

Blood Sugar Log	Before	After	Insulin
Breakfast			
Lunch			
Dinner			
Bedtime			

Note

____

____

Mood

Date____/____/____   Day:______   MO TU WE TH FR SA SU

Daily Food and Beverage Log

Food	BREAKFAST				
	Cals	Carbs	Fiber	Protein	Sugar
MEAL SUBTOTAL					

Food	LUNCH				
	Cals	Carbs	Fiber	Protein	Sugar
MEAL SUBTOTAL					

Food	DINNER				
	Cals	Carbs	Fiber	Protein	Sugar
MEAL SUBTOTAL					

Food	SNACKS				
	Cals	Carbs	Fiber	Protein	Sugar
MEAL SUBTOTAL					

DAILY GRAND TOTAL	Cals	Carbs	Fiber	Protein	Sugar	Met my goals today?	Yes	No

WORKOUT LOG

The exercise program and provides.

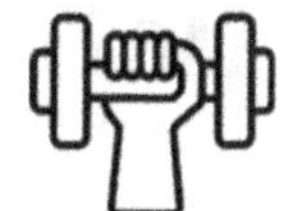

WEIGHT:	
SLEEP (hrs):	
CALORIES:	
TIME (minutes):	

EXERCISES	SETS	Duration	Intensity	Cal/Burn

Blood Sugar Log	Before	After	Insulin
Breakfast			
Lunch			
Dinner			
Bedtime			

Note

Mood

Date ___/___/___   Day: ______   MO TU WE TH FR SA SU

Daily Food and Beverage Log

Food	BREAKFAST				
	Cals	Carbs	Fiber	Protein	Sugar
MEAL SUBTOTAL					

Food	LUNCH				
	Cals	Carbs	Fiber	Protein	Sugar
MEAL SUBTOTAL					

Food	DINNER				
	Cals	Carbs	Fiber	Protein	Sugar
MEAL SUBTOTAL					

Food	SNACKS				
	Cals	Carbs	Fiber	Protein	Sugar
MEAL SUBTOTAL					

DAILY GRAND TOTAL	Cals	Carbs	Fiber	Protein	Sugar	Met my goals today?	Yes	No

WORKOUT LOG

The exercise program and provides.

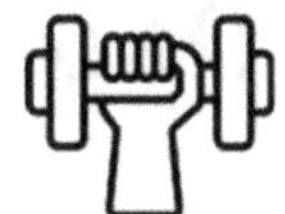

WEIGHT:	
SLEEP (hrs):	
CALORIES:	
TIME (minutes):	

EXERCISES	SETS	Duration	Intensity	Cal/Burn

Blood Sugar Log	Before	After	Insulin
Breakfast			
Lunch			
Dinner			
Bedtime			

Note

Mood

Date____/____/____ Day:______ MO TU WE TH FR SA SU

Daily Food and Beverage Log

Food	BREAKFAST				
	Cals	Carbs	Fiber	Protein	Sugar
MEAL SUBTOTAL					

Food	LUNCH				
	Cals	Carbs	Fiber	Protein	Sugar
MEAL SUBTOTAL					

Food	DINNER				
	Cals	Carbs	Fiber	Protein	Sugar
MEAL SUBTOTAL					

Food	SNACKS				
	Cals	Carbs	Fiber	Protein	Sugar
MEAL SUBTOTAL					

DAILY GRAND TOTAL	Cals	Carbs	Fiber	Protein	Sugar	Met my goals today?	Yes	No

WORKOUT LOG

The exercise program and provides.

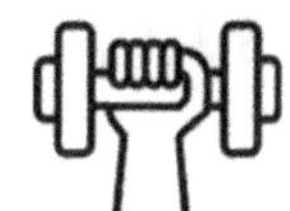

WEIGHT:	
SLEEP (hrs):	
CALORIES:	
TIME (minutes):	

EXERCISES	SETS	Duration	Intensity	Cal/Burn

Blood Sugar Log	Before	After	Insulin
Breakfast			
Lunch			
Dinner			
Bedtime			

Note

Mood

Daily Food and Beverage Log

Date______/______/______   Day: ________   MO TU WE TH FR SA SU

Food		BREAKFAST				
		Cals	Carbs	Fiber	Protein	Sugar
MEAL SUBTOTAL						

Food		LUNCH				
		Cals	Carbs	Fiber	Protein	Sugar
MEAL SUBTOTAL						

Food		DINNER				
		Cals	Carbs	Fiber	Protein	Sugar
MEAL SUBTOTAL						

Food		SNACKS				
		Cals	Carbs	Fiber	Protein	Sugar
MEAL SUBTOTAL						

DAILY GRAND TOTAL	Cals	Carbs	Fiber	Protein	Sugar	Met my goals today?	Yes	No

WORKOUT LOG

The exercise program and provides.

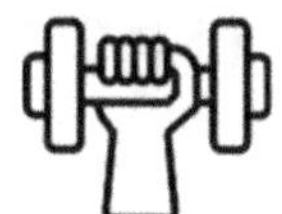

WEIGHT:	
SLEEP (hrs):	
CALORIES:	
TIME (minutes):	

EXERCISES	SETS	Duration	Intensity	Cal/Burn

Blood Sugar Log	Before	After	Insulin
Breakfast			
Lunch			
Dinner			
Bedtime			

Note

Mood

Date_____ / _____ / _____   Day: _______   MO TU WE TH FR SA SU

Daily Food and Beverage Log

Food	BREAKFAST				
	Cals	Carbs	Fiber	Protein	Sugar
MEAL SUBTOTAL					

Food	LUNCH				
	Cals	Carbs	Fiber	Protein	Sugar
MEAL SUBTOTAL					

Food	DINNER				
	Cals	Carbs	Fiber	Protein	Sugar
MEAL SUBTOTAL					

Food	SNACKS				
	Cals	Carbs	Fiber	Protein	Sugar
MEAL SUBTOTAL					

DAILY GRAND TOTAL	Cals	Carbs	Fiber	Protein	Sugar	Met my goals today?	Yes	No

WORKOUT LOG

The exercise program and provides.

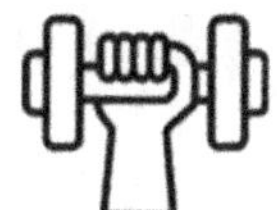

WEIGHT:	
SLEEP (hrs):	
CALORIES:	
TIME (minutes):	

Vitamin/ Supplements/ Meds

....

....

....

EXERCISES	SETS	Duration	Intensity	Cal/Burn

Blood Sugar Log	Before	After	Insulin
Breakfast			
Lunch			
Dinner			
Bedtime			

Note

____

____

Mood

Date___/___/___   Day: _______   MO TU WE TH FR SA SU

Daily Food and Beverage Log

Food	BREAKFAST				
	Cals	Carbs	Fiber	Protein	Sugar
MEAL SUBTOTAL					

Food	LUNCH				
	Cals	Carbs	Fiber	Protein	Sugar
MEAL SUBTOTAL					

Food	DINNER				
	Cals	Carbs	Fiber	Protein	Sugar
MEAL SUBTOTAL					

Food	SNACKS				
	Cals	Carbs	Fiber	Protein	Sugar
MEAL SUBTOTAL					

DAILY GRAND TOTAL	Cals	Carbs	Fiber	Protein	Sugar	Met my goals today?	Yes	No

WORKOUT LOG

The exercise program and provides.

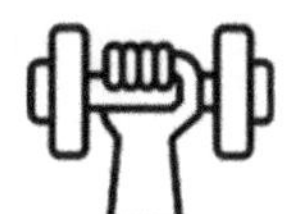

WEIGHT:	
SLEEP (hrs):	
CALORIES:	
TIME (minutes):	

Vitamin/ Supplements/ Meds

EXERCISES	SETS	Duration	Intensity	Cal/Burn

Blood Sugar Log	Before	After	Insulin
Breakfast			
Lunch			
Dinner			
Bedtime			

Note

Mood

Daily Food and Beverage Log

Date____ / ____ / ____   Day: ______   MO TU WE TH FR SA SU

Food	BREAKFAST				
	Cals	Carbs	Fiber	Protein	Sugar
MEAL SUBTOTAL					

Food	LUNCH				
	Cals	Carbs	Fiber	Protein	Sugar
MEAL SUBTOTAL					

Food	DINNER				
	Cals	Carbs	Fiber	Protein	Sugar
MEAL SUBTOTAL					

Food	SNACKS				
	Cals	Carbs	Fiber	Protein	Sugar
MEAL SUBTOTAL					

DAILY GRAND TOTAL	Cals	Carbs	Fiber	Protein	Sugar	Met my goals today?	Yes	No

WORKOUT LOG

The exercise program and provides.

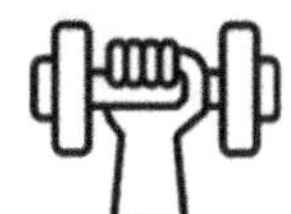

WEIGHT:	
SLEEP (hrs):	
CALORIES:	
TIME (minutes):	

EXERCISES	SETS	Duration	Intensity	Cal/Burn

Blood Sugar Log	Before	After	Insulin
Breakfast			
Lunch			
Dinner			
Bedtime			

Note

Mood

Date____/____/____ Day:______   MO TU WE TH FR SA SU

Daily Food and Beverage Log

Food	BREAKFAST				
	Cals	Carbs	Fiber	Protein	Sugar
MEAL SUBTOTAL					

Food	LUNCH				
	Cals	Carbs	Fiber	Protein	Sugar
MEAL SUBTOTAL					

Food	DINNER				
	Cals	Carbs	Fiber	Protein	Sugar
MEAL SUBTOTAL					

Food	SNACKS				
	Cals	Carbs	Fiber	Protein	Sugar
MEAL SUBTOTAL					

DAILY GRAND TOTAL	Cals	Carbs	Fiber	Protein	Sugar	Met my goals today?	Yes	No

WORKOUT LOG

The exercise program and provides.

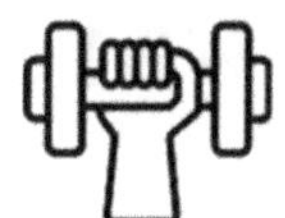

WEIGHT:	
SLEEP (hrs):	
CALORIES:	
TIME (minutes):	

EXERCISES	SETS	Duration	Intensity	Cal/Burn

Blood Sugar Log	Before	After	Insulin
Breakfast			
Lunch			
Dinner			
Bedtime			

Note

Mood

Date____ / ____ / ____   Day: ______   MO TU WE TH FR SA SU

Daily Food and Beverage Log

Food	BREAKFAST				
	Cals	Carbs	Fiber	Protein	Sugar
MEAL SUBTOTAL					

Food	LUNCH				
	Cals	Carbs	Fiber	Protein	Sugar
MEAL SUBTOTAL					

Food	DINNER				
	Cals	Carbs	Fiber	Protein	Sugar
MEAL SUBTOTAL					

Food	SNACKS				
	Cals	Carbs	Fiber	Protein	Sugar
MEAL SUBTOTAL					

DAILY GRAND TOTAL	Cals	Carbs	Fiber	Protein	Sugar	Met my goals today?	Yes	No

WORKOUT LOG

The exercise program and provides.

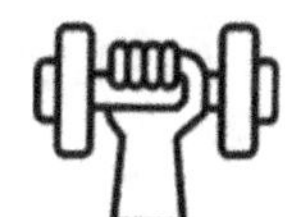

WEIGHT:	
SLEEP (hrs):	
CALORIES:	
TIME (minutes):	

EXERCISES	SETS	Duration	Intensity	Cal/Burn

Blood Sugar Log	Before	After	Insulin
Breakfast			
Lunch			
Dinner			
Bedtime			

Note

Mood

Date______/____/______   Day: ______   MO TU WE TH FR SA SU

Daily Food and Beverage Log

Food	BREAKFAST				
	Cals	Carbs	Fiber	Protein	Sugar
MEAL SUBTOTAL					

Food	LUNCH				
	Cals	Carbs	Fiber	Protein	Sugar
MEAL SUBTOTAL					

Food	DINNER				
	Cals	Carbs	Fiber	Protein	Sugar
MEAL SUBTOTAL					

Food	SNACKS				
	Cals	Carbs	Fiber	Protein	Sugar
MEAL SUBTOTAL					

DAILY GRAND TOTAL	Cals	Carbs	Fiber	Protein	Sugar	Met my goals today?	Yes	No

WORKOUT LOG

The exercise program and provides.

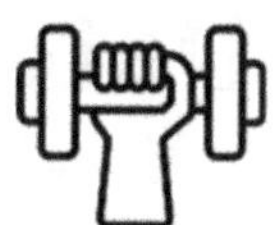

WEIGHT:	
SLEEP (hrs):	
CALORIES:	
TIME (minutes):	

EXERCISES	SETS	Duration	Intensity	Cal/Burn

Blood Sugar Log	Before	After	Insulin
Breakfast			
Lunch			
Dinner			
Bedtime			

Note

Mood

Date____/____/____   Day:______   MO TU WE TH FR SA SU

Daily Food and Beverage Log

Food	BREAKFAST				
	Cals	Carbs	Fiber	Protein	Sugar
MEAL SUBTOTAL					

Food	LUNCH				
	Cals	Carbs	Fiber	Protein	Sugar
MEAL SUBTOTAL					

Food	DINNER				
	Cals	Carbs	Fiber	Protein	Sugar
MEAL SUBTOTAL					

Food	SNACKS				
	Cals	Carbs	Fiber	Protein	Sugar
MEAL SUBTOTAL					

DAILY GRAND TOTAL	Cals	Carbs	Fiber	Protein	Sugar	Met my goals today?	Yes	No

WORKOUT LOG

The exercise program and provides.

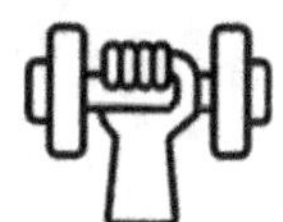

WEIGHT:	
SLEEP (hrs):	
CALORIES:	
TIME (minutes):	

Vitamin / Supplements / Meds

....

....

....

EXERCISES	SETS	Duration	Intensity	Cal/Burn

Blood Sugar Log	Before	After	Insulin
Breakfast			
Lunch			
Dinner			
Bedtime			

Note

____

____

Mood

Date_____/_____/_____   Day: _______   MO TU WE TH FR SA SU

Daily Food and Beverage Log

Food	BREAKFAST				
	Cals	Carbs	Fiber	Protein	Sugar
MEAL SUBTOTAL					

Food	LUNCH				
	Cals	Carbs	Fiber	Protein	Sugar
MEAL SUBTOTAL					

Food	DINNER				
	Cals	Carbs	Fiber	Protein	Sugar
MEAL SUBTOTAL					

Food	SNACKS				
	Cals	Carbs	Fiber	Protein	Sugar
MEAL SUBTOTAL					

DAILY GRAND TOTAL	Cals	Carbs	Fiber	Protein	Sugar	Met my goals today?	Yes	No

WORKOUT LOG

The exercise program and provides.

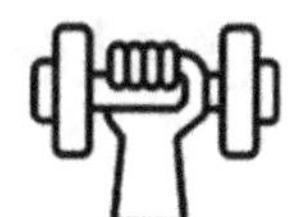

WEIGHT:	
SLEEP (hrs):	
CALORIES:	
TIME (minutes):	

EXERCISES	SETS	Duration	Intensity	Cal/Burn

Blood Sugar Log	Before	After	Insulin
Breakfast			
Lunch			
Dinner			
Bedtime			

Note

Mood

Daily Food and Beverage Log

Date______/______/______   Day:_______   MO TU WE TH FR SA SU

Food	BREAKFAST				
	Cals	Carbs	Fiber	Protein	Sugar
MEAL SUBTOTAL					

Food	LUNCH				
	Cals	Carbs	Fiber	Protein	Sugar
MEAL SUBTOTAL					

Food	DINNER				
	Cals	Carbs	Fiber	Protein	Sugar
MEAL SUBTOTAL					

Food	SNACKS				
	Cals	Carbs	Fiber	Protein	Sugar
MEAL SUBTOTAL					

DAILY GRAND TOTAL	Cals	Carbs	Fiber	Protein	Sugar	Met my goals today?	Yes	No

WORKOUT LOG

The exercise program and provides.

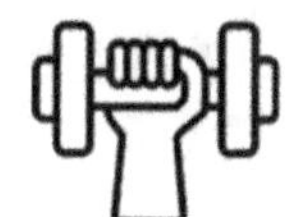

WEIGHT:	
SLEEP (hrs):	
CALORIES:	
TIME (minutes):	

EXERCISES	SETS	Duration	Intensity	Cal/Burn

Blood Sugar Log	Before	After	Insulin
Breakfast			
Lunch			
Dinner			
Bedtime			

Note

Mood

Daily Food and Beverage Log

Date_______/_____/______   Day:________   MO TU WE TH FR SA SU

Food	BREAKFAST				
	Cals	Carbs	Fiber	Protein	Sugar
MEAL SUBTOTAL					

Food	LUNCH				
	Cals	Carbs	Fiber	Protein	Sugar
MEAL SUBTOTAL					

Food	DINNER				
	Cals	Carbs	Fiber	Protein	Sugar
MEAL SUBTOTAL					

Food	SNACKS				
	Cals	Carbs	Fiber	Protein	Sugar
MEAL SUBTOTAL					

DAILY GRAND TOTAL	Cals	Carbs	Fiber	Protein	Sugar	Met my goals today?	Yes	No

WORKOUT LOG

The exercise program and provides.

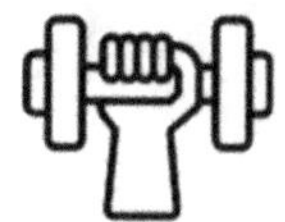

WEIGHT:	
SLEEP (hrs):	
CALORIES:	
TIME (minutes):	

EXERCISES	SETS	Duration	Intensity	Cal/Burn

Blood Sugar Log	Before	After	Insulin
Breakfast			
Lunch			
Dinner			
Bedtime			

Note

Mood

Date___/___/___   Day: ______   MO TU WE TH FR SA SU

Daily Food and Beverage Log

Food	BREAKFAST				
	Cals	Carbs	Fiber	Protein	Sugar
MEAL SUBTOTAL					

Food	LUNCH				
	Cals	Carbs	Fiber	Protein	Sugar
MEAL SUBTOTAL					

Food	DINNER				
	Cals	Carbs	Fiber	Protein	Sugar
MEAL SUBTOTAL					

Food	SNACKS				
	Cals	Carbs	Fiber	Protein	Sugar
MEAL SUBTOTAL					

DAILY GRAND TOTAL	Cals	Carbs	Fiber	Protein	Sugar	Met my goals today?	Yes	No

WORKOUT LOG

The exercise program and provides.

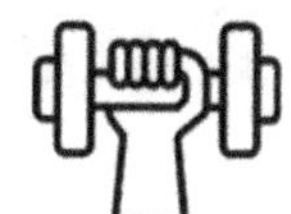

WEIGHT:	
SLEEP (hrs):	
CALORIES:	
TIME (minutes):	

EXERCISES	SETS	Duration	Intensity	Cal/Burn

Blood Sugar Log	Before	After	Insulin
Breakfast			
Lunch			
Dinner			
Bedtime			

Note

Mood

Date_____/_____/_____   Day:_______   MO TU WE TH FR SA SU

Daily Food and Beverage Log

Food	BREAKFAST				
	Cals	Carbs	Fiber	Protein	Sugar
MEAL SUBTOTAL					

Food	LUNCH				
	Cals	Carbs	Fiber	Protein	Sugar
MEAL SUBTOTAL					

Food	DINNER				
	Cals	Carbs	Fiber	Protein	Sugar
MEAL SUBTOTAL					

Food	SNACKS				
	Cals	Carbs	Fiber	Protein	Sugar
MEAL SUBTOTAL					

DAILY GRAND TOTAL	Cals	Carbs	Fiber	Protein	Sugar	Met my goals today?	Yes	No

WORKOUT LOG

The exercise program and provides.

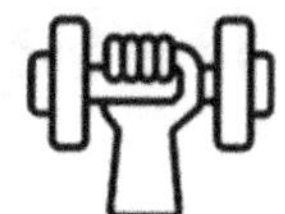

WEIGHT:	
SLEEP (hrs):	
CALORIES:	
TIME (minutes):	

EXERCISES	SETS	Duration	Intensity	Cal/Burn

Blood Sugar Log	Before	After	Insulin
Breakfast			
Lunch			
Dinner			
Bedtime			

Note

Mood

Date____/____/____   Day:______   MO TU WE TH FR SA SU

Daily Food and Beverage Log

Food	BREAKFAST				
	Cals	Carbs	Fiber	Protein	Sugar
MEAL SUBTOTAL					

Food	LUNCH				
	Cals	Carbs	Fiber	Protein	Sugar
MEAL SUBTOTAL					

Food	DINNER				
	Cals	Carbs	Fiber	Protein	Sugar
MEAL SUBTOTAL					

Food	SNACKS				
	Cals	Carbs	Fiber	Protein	Sugar
MEAL SUBTOTAL					

DAILY GRAND TOTAL	Cals	Carbs	Fiber	Protein	Sugar	Met my goals today?	Yes	No

WORKOUT LOG

The exercise program and provides.

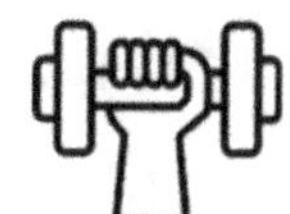

WEIGHT:	
SLEEP (hrs):	
CALORIES:	
TIME (minutes):	

Vitamin/ Supplements/ Meds

....

....

....

EXERCISES	SETS	Duration	Intensity	Cal/Burn

Blood Sugar Log	Before	After	Insulin
Breakfast			
Lunch			
Dinner			
Bedtime			

Note

____

____

Mood

Daily Food and Beverage Log

Date______/______/______   Day: ________   MO TU WE TH FR SA SU

Food	BREAKFAST				
	Cals	Carbs	Fiber	Protein	Sugar
MEAL SUBTOTAL					

Food	LUNCH				
	Cals	Carbs	Fiber	Protein	Sugar
MEAL SUBTOTAL					

Food	DINNER				
	Cals	Carbs	Fiber	Protein	Sugar
MEAL SUBTOTAL					

Food	SNACKS				
	Cals	Carbs	Fiber	Protein	Sugar
MEAL SUBTOTAL					

DAILY GRAND TOTAL	Cals	Carbs	Fiber	Protein	Sugar	Met my goals today?	Yes	No

WORKOUT LOG

The exercise program and provides.

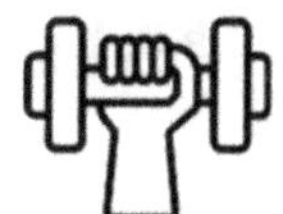

WEIGHT:	
SLEEP (hrs):	
CALORIES:	
TIME (minutes):	

Vitamin / Supplements / Meds

....

....

....

EXERCISES	SETS	Duration	Intensity	Cal/Burn

Blood Sugar Log	Before	After	Insulin
Breakfast			
Lunch			
Dinner			
Bedtime			

Note

____

____

Mood

Date ___/___/___   Day: _____   MO TU WE TH FR SA SU

Daily Food and Beverage Log

Food	BREAKFAST				
	Cals	Carbs	Fiber	Protein	Sugar
MEAL SUBTOTAL					

Food	LUNCH				
	Cals	Carbs	Fiber	Protein	Sugar
MEAL SUBTOTAL					

Food	DINNER				
	Cals	Carbs	Fiber	Protein	Sugar
MEAL SUBTOTAL					

Food	SNACKS				
	Cals	Carbs	Fiber	Protein	Sugar
MEAL SUBTOTAL					

DAILY GRAND TOTAL	Cals	Carbs	Fiber	Protein	Sugar	Met my goals today?	Yes	No

WORKOUT LOG

The exercise program and provides.

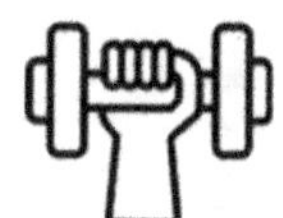

WEIGHT:	
SLEEP (hrs):	
CALORIES:	
TIME (minutes):	

Vitamin/ Supplements/ Meds

....

....

....

EXERCISES	SETS	Duration	Intensity	Cal/Burn

Blood Sugar Log	Before	After	Insulin
Breakfast			
Lunch			
Dinner			
Bedtime			

Note

____

____

Mood

Daily Food and Beverage Log

Date____/____/____   Day:______   MO TU WE TH FR SA SU

Food	BREAKFAST				
	Cals	Carbs	Fiber	Protein	Sugar
MEAL SUBTOTAL					

Food	LUNCH				
	Cals	Carbs	Fiber	Protein	Sugar
MEAL SUBTOTAL					

Food	DINNER				
	Cals	Carbs	Fiber	Protein	Sugar
MEAL SUBTOTAL					

Food	SNACKS				
	Cals	Carbs	Fiber	Protein	Sugar
MEAL SUBTOTAL					

DAILY GRAND TOTAL	Cals	Carbs	Fiber	Protein	Sugar	Met my goals today?	Yes	No

WORKOUT LOG

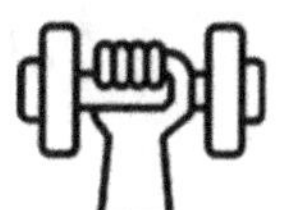

The exercise program and provides.

WEIGHT:	
SLEEP (hrs):	
CALORIES:	
TIME (minutes):	

Vitamin/ Supplements/ Meds

EXERCISES	SETS	Duration	Intensity	Cal/Burn

Blood Sugar Log	Before	After	Insulin
Breakfast			
Lunch			
Dinner			
Bedtime			

Note

Mood

Date ____/____/____   Day: ______   MO TU WE TH FR SA SU

Daily Food and Beverage Log

Food	BREAKFAST				
	Cals	Carbs	Fiber	Protein	Sugar
MEAL SUBTOTAL					

Food	LUNCH				
	Cals	Carbs	Fiber	Protein	Sugar
MEAL SUBTOTAL					

Food	DINNER				
	Cals	Carbs	Fiber	Protein	Sugar
MEAL SUBTOTAL					

Food	SNACKS				
	Cals	Carbs	Fiber	Protein	Sugar
MEAL SUBTOTAL					

DAILY GRAND TOTAL	Cals	Carbs	Fiber	Protein	Sugar	Met my goals today?	Yes	No

WORKOUT LOG

The exercise program and provides.

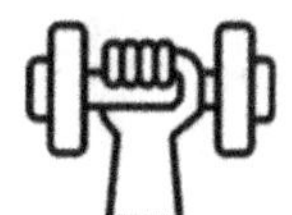

WEIGHT:	
SLEEP (hrs):	
CALORIES:	
TIME (minutes):	

EXERCISES	SETS	Duration	Intensity	Cal/Burn

Blood Sugar Log	Before	After	Insulin
Breakfast			
Lunch			
Dinner			
Bedtime			

Note

Mood

Date ___/___/___   Day: ______   MO TU WE TH FR SA SU

Daily Food and Beverage Log

Food	BREAKFAST				
	Cals	Carbs	Fiber	Protein	Sugar
MEAL SUBTOTAL					

Food	LUNCH				
	Cals	Carbs	Fiber	Protein	Sugar
MEAL SUBTOTAL					

Food	DINNER				
	Cals	Carbs	Fiber	Protein	Sugar
MEAL SUBTOTAL					

Food	SNACKS				
	Cals	Carbs	Fiber	Protein	Sugar
MEAL SUBTOTAL					

DAILY GRAND TOTAL	Cals	Carbs	Fiber	Protein	Sugar	Met my goals today?	Yes	No

WORKOUT LOG

The exercise program and provides.

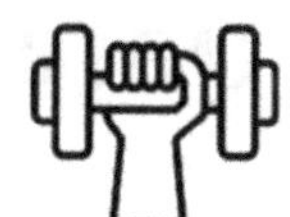

WEIGHT:	
SLEEP (hrs):	
CALORIES:	
TIME (minutes):	

EXERCISES	SETS	Duration	Intensity	Cal/Burn

Blood Sugar Log	Before	After	Insulin
Breakfast			
Lunch			
Dinner			
Bedtime			

Note

Mood

Daily Food and Beverage Log

Date_____/_____/_____   Day:_______   MO TU WE TH FR SA SU

Food	BREAKFAST				
	Cals	Carbs	Fiber	Protein	Sugar
MEAL SUBTOTAL					

Food	LUNCH				
	Cals	Carbs	Fiber	Protein	Sugar
MEAL SUBTOTAL					

Food	DINNER				
	Cals	Carbs	Fiber	Protein	Sugar
MEAL SUBTOTAL					

Food	SNACKS				
	Cals	Carbs	Fiber	Protein	Sugar
MEAL SUBTOTAL					

DAILY GRAND TOTAL	Cals	Carbs	Fiber	Protein	Sugar	Met my goals today?	Yes	No

WORKOUT LOG

The exercise program and provides.

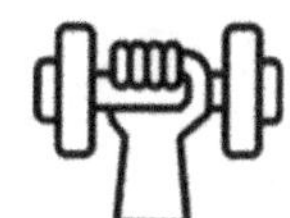

WEIGHT:	
SLEEP (hrs):	
CALORIES:	
TIME (minutes):	

EXERCISES	SETS	Duration	Intensity	Cal/Burn

Blood Sugar Log	Before	After	Insulin
Breakfast			
Lunch			
Dinner			
Bedtime			

Note

____

____

Mood

Date____/____/____ Day: ______ MO TU WE TH FR SA SU

Daily Food and Beverage Log

Food	BREAKFAST				
	Cals	Carbs	Fiber	Protein	Sugar
MEAL SUBTOTAL					

Food	LUNCH				
	Cals	Carbs	Fiber	Protein	Sugar
MEAL SUBTOTAL					

Food	DINNER				
	Cals	Carbs	Fiber	Protein	Sugar
MEAL SUBTOTAL					

Food	SNACKS				
	Cals	Carbs	Fiber	Protein	Sugar
MEAL SUBTOTAL					

DAILY GRAND TOTAL	Cals	Carbs	Fiber	Protein	Sugar	Met my goals today?	Yes	No

WORKOUT LOG

The exercise program and provides.

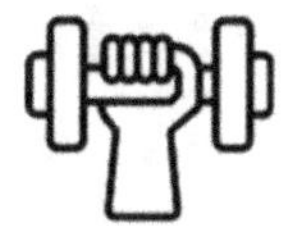

WEIGHT:	
SLEEP (hrs):	
CALORIES:	
TIME (minutes):	

Vitamin/ Supplements/ Meds

....

....

....

EXERCISES	SETS	Duration	Intensity	Cal/Burn

Blood Sugar Log	Before	After	Insulin
Breakfast			
Lunch			
Dinner			
Bedtime			

Note

____

____

Mood

Date____/___/____ Day:______ MO TU WE TH FR SA SU

Daily Food and Beverage Log

Food	BREAKFAST				
	Cals	Carbs	Fiber	Protein	Sugar
MEAL SUBTOTAL					

Food	LUNCH				
	Cals	Carbs	Fiber	Protein	Sugar
MEAL SUBTOTAL					

Food	DINNER				
	Cals	Carbs	Fiber	Protein	Sugar
MEAL SUBTOTAL					

Food	SNACKS				
	Cals	Carbs	Fiber	Protein	Sugar
MEAL SUBTOTAL					

DAILY GRAND TOTAL	Cals	Carbs	Fiber	Protein	Sugar	Met my goals today?	Yes	No

WORKOUT LOG

The exercise program and provides.

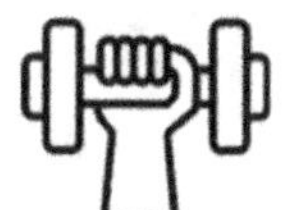

WEIGHT:	
SLEEP (hrs):	
CALORIES:	
TIME (minutes):	

EXERCISES	SETS	Duration	Intensity	Cal/Burn

Blood Sugar Log	Before	After	Insulin
Breakfast			
Lunch			
Dinner			
Bedtime			

Note

Mood

Daily Food and Beverage Log

Food	BREAKFAST				
	Cals	Carbs	Fiber	Protein	Sugar
MEAL SUBTOTAL					

Food	LUNCH				
	Cals	Carbs	Fiber	Protein	Sugar
MEAL SUBTOTAL					

Food	DINNER				
	Cals	Carbs	Fiber	Protein	Sugar
MEAL SUBTOTAL					

Food	SNACKS				
	Cals	Carbs	Fiber	Protein	Sugar
MEAL SUBTOTAL					

DAILY GRAND TOTAL	Cals	Carbs	Fiber	Protein	Sugar	Met my goals today?	Yes	No

WORKOUT LOG

The exercise program and provides.

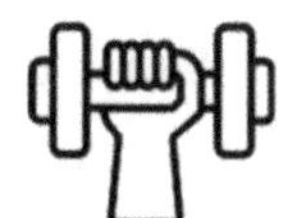

WEIGHT:	
SLEEP (hrs):	
CALORIES:	
TIME (minutes):	

EXERCISES	SETS	Duration	Intensity	Cal/Burn

Blood Sugar Log	Before	After	Insulin
Breakfast			
Lunch			
Dinner			
Bedtime			

Note

Mood

Date_____/_____/_____ Day:______ MO TU WE TH FR SA SU

Daily Food and Beverage Log

Food	BREAKFAST				
	Cals	Carbs	Fiber	Protein	Sugar
MEAL SUBTOTAL					

Food	LUNCH				
	Cals	Carbs	Fiber	Protein	Sugar
MEAL SUBTOTAL					

Food	DINNER				
	Cals	Carbs	Fiber	Protein	Sugar
MEAL SUBTOTAL					

Food	SNACKS				
	Cals	Carbs	Fiber	Protein	Sugar
MEAL SUBTOTAL					

DAILY GRAND TOTAL	Cals	Carbs	Fiber	Protein	Sugar	Met my goals today?	Yes	No

WORKOUT LOG

The exercise program and provides.

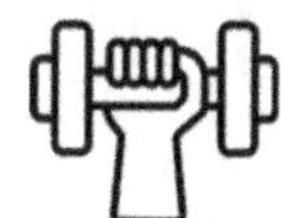

WEIGHT:	
SLEEP (hrs):	
CALORIES:	
TIME (minutes):	

EXERCISES	SETS	Duration	Intensity	Cal/Burn

Blood Sugar Log	Before	After	Insulin
Breakfast			
Lunch			
Dinner			
Bedtime			

Note

Mood

Date_____ / _____ / _____   Day: ______   MO TU WE TH FR SA SU

Daily Food and Beverage Log

Food	BREAKFAST				
	Cals	Carbs	Fiber	Protein	Sugar
MEAL SUBTOTAL					

Food	LUNCH				
	Cals	Carbs	Fiber	Protein	Sugar
MEAL SUBTOTAL					

Food	DINNER				
	Cals	Carbs	Fiber	Protein	Sugar
MEAL SUBTOTAL					

Food	SNACKS				
	Cals	Carbs	Fiber	Protein	Sugar
MEAL SUBTOTAL					

DAILY GRAND TOTAL	Cals	Carbs	Fiber	Protein	Sugar	Met my goals today?	Yes	No

WORKOUT LOG

The exercise program and provides.

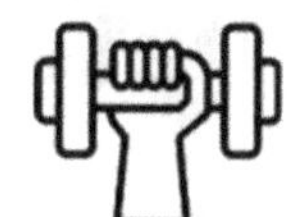

WEIGHT:	
SLEEP (hrs):	
CALORIES:	
TIME (minutes):	

EXERCISES	SETS	Duration	Intensity	Cal/Burn

Blood Sugar Log	Before	After	Insulin
Breakfast			
Lunch			
Dinner			
Bedtime			

Note

Mood

Date___/___/___   Day:______   MO TU WE TH FR SA SU

Daily Food and Beverage Log

Food	BREAKFAST				
	Cals	Carbs	Fiber	Protein	Sugar
MEAL SUBTOTAL					

Food	LUNCH				
	Cals	Carbs	Fiber	Protein	Sugar
MEAL SUBTOTAL					

Food	DINNER				
	Cals	Carbs	Fiber	Protein	Sugar
MEAL SUBTOTAL					

Food	SNACKS				
	Cals	Carbs	Fiber	Protein	Sugar
MEAL SUBTOTAL					

DAILY GRAND TOTAL	Cals	Carbs	Fiber	Protein	Sugar	Met my goals today?	Yes	No

WORKOUT LOG

The exercise program and provides.

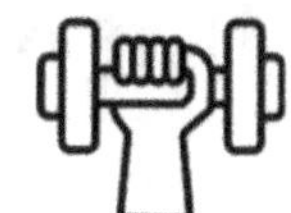

WEIGHT:	
SLEEP (hrs):	
CALORIES:	
TIME (minutes):	

Vitamin/ Supplements/ Meds

....

....

....

EXERCISES	SETS	Duration	Intensity	Cal/Burn

Blood Sugar Log	Before	After	Insulin
Breakfast			
Lunch			
Dinner			
Bedtime			

Note

____

____

Mood

Daily Food and Beverage Log

Date______/______/______ Day:________ MO TU WE TH FR SA SU

Food	BREAKFAST				
	Cals	Carbs	Fiber	Protein	Sugar
MEAL SUBTOTAL					

Food	LUNCH				
	Cals	Carbs	Fiber	Protein	Sugar
MEAL SUBTOTAL					

Food	DINNER				
	Cals	Carbs	Fiber	Protein	Sugar
MEAL SUBTOTAL					

Food	SNACKS				
	Cals	Carbs	Fiber	Protein	Sugar
MEAL SUBTOTAL					

DAILY GRAND TOTAL	Cals	Carbs	Fiber	Protein	Sugar	Met my goals today?	Yes	No

WORKOUT LOG

The exercise program and provides.

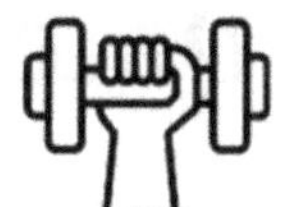

WEIGHT:	
SLEEP (hrs):	
CALORIES:	
TIME (minutes):	

EXERCISES	SETS	Duration	Intensity	Cal/Burn

Blood Sugar Log	Before	After	Insulin
Breakfast			
Lunch			
Dinner			
Bedtime			

Note

____

____

Mood

Date____/____/____   Day:______   MO TU WE TH FR SA SU

Daily Food and Beverage Log

Food	BREAKFAST				
	Cals	Carbs	Fiber	Protein	Sugar
MEAL SUBTOTAL					

Food	LUNCH				
	Cals	Carbs	Fiber	Protein	Sugar
MEAL SUBTOTAL					

Food	DINNER				
	Cals	Carbs	Fiber	Protein	Sugar
MEAL SUBTOTAL					

Food	SNACKS				
	Cals	Carbs	Fiber	Protein	Sugar
MEAL SUBTOTAL					

DAILY GRAND TOTAL	Cals	Carbs	Fiber	Protein	Sugar	Met my goals today?	Yes	No

WORKOUT LOG

The exercise program and provides.

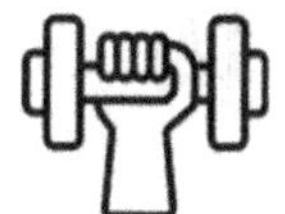

WEIGHT:	
SLEEP (hrs):	
CALORIES:	
TIME (minutes):	

EXERCISES	SETS	Duration	Intensity	Cal/Burn

Blood Sugar Log	Before	After	Insulin
Breakfast			
Lunch			
Dinner			
Bedtime			

Note

Mood

Date____/____/____   Day: ______   MO TU WE TH FR SA SU

Daily Food and Beverage Log

Food	BREAKFAST				
	Cals	Carbs	Fiber	Protein	Sugar
MEAL SUBTOTAL					

Food	LUNCH				
	Cals	Carbs	Fiber	Protein	Sugar
MEAL SUBTOTAL					

Food	DINNER				
	Cals	Carbs	Fiber	Protein	Sugar
MEAL SUBTOTAL					

Food	SNACKS				
	Cals	Carbs	Fiber	Protein	Sugar
MEAL SUBTOTAL					

DAILY GRAND TOTAL	Cals	Carbs	Fiber	Protein	Sugar	Met my goals today?	Yes	No

WORKOUT LOG

The exercise program and provides.

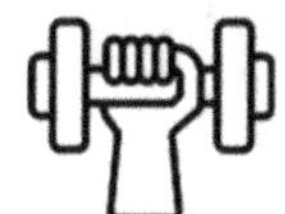

WEIGHT:	
SLEEP (hrs):	
CALORIES:	
TIME (minutes):	

Vitamin/ Supplements/ Meds

....

....

....

EXERCISES	SETS	Duration	Intensity	Cal/Burn

Blood Sugar Log	Before	After	Insulin
Breakfast			
Lunch			
Dinner			
Bedtime			

Note

____

____

Mood

Daily Food and Beverage Log

Date______/______/______   Day: ______   MO TU WE TH FR SA SU

Food	BREAKFAST				
	Cals	Carbs	Fiber	Protein	Sugar
MEAL SUBTOTAL					

Food	LUNCH				
	Cals	Carbs	Fiber	Protein	Sugar
MEAL SUBTOTAL					

Food	DINNER				
	Cals	Carbs	Fiber	Protein	Sugar
MEAL SUBTOTAL					

Food	SNACKS				
	Cals	Carbs	Fiber	Protein	Sugar
MEAL SUBTOTAL					

DAILY GRAND TOTAL	Cals	Carbs	Fiber	Protein	Sugar	Met my goals today?	Yes	No

WORKOUT LOG

The exercise program and provides.

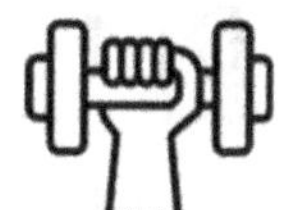

WEIGHT:	
SLEEP (hrs):	
CALORIES:	
TIME (minutes):	

Vitamin / Supplements / Meds

EXERCISES	SETS	Duration	Intensity	Cal/Burn

Blood Sugar Log	Before	After	Insulin
Breakfast			
Lunch			
Dinner			
Bedtime			

Note

Mood

Date_____/_____/_____   Day:______   MO TU WE TH FR SA SU

Daily Food and Beverage Log

Food	BREAKFAST				
	Cals	Carbs	Fiber	Protein	Sugar
MEAL SUBTOTAL					

Food	LUNCH				
	Cals	Carbs	Fiber	Protein	Sugar
MEAL SUBTOTAL					

Food	DINNER				
	Cals	Carbs	Fiber	Protein	Sugar
MEAL SUBTOTAL					

Food	SNACKS				
	Cals	Carbs	Fiber	Protein	Sugar
MEAL SUBTOTAL					

DAILY GRAND TOTAL	Cals	Carbs	Fiber	Protein	Sugar	Met my goals today?	Yes	No

WORKOUT LOG

The exercise program and provides.

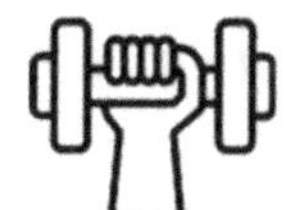

WEIGHT:	
SLEEP (hrs):	
CALORIES:	
TIME (minutes):	

Vitamin/ Supplements/ Meds

....

....

....

EXERCISES	SETS	Duration	Intensity	Cal/Burn

Blood Sugar Log	Before	After	Insulin
Breakfast			
Lunch			
Dinner			
Bedtime			

Note

____

____

Mood

Date____/____/____   Day:______   MO TU WE TH FR SA SU

Daily Food and Beverage Log

Food	BREAKFAST				
	Cals	Carbs	Fiber	Protein	Sugar
MEAL SUBTOTAL					

Food	LUNCH				
	Cals	Carbs	Fiber	Protein	Sugar
MEAL SUBTOTAL					

Food	DINNER				
	Cals	Carbs	Fiber	Protein	Sugar
MEAL SUBTOTAL					

Food	SNACKS				
	Cals	Carbs	Fiber	Protein	Sugar
MEAL SUBTOTAL					

DAILY GRAND TOTAL	Cals	Carbs	Fiber	Protein	Sugar	Met my goals today?	Yes	No

WORKOUT LOG

The exercise program and provides.

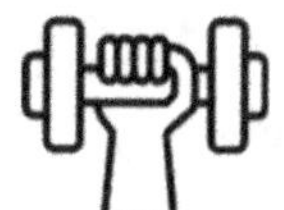

WEIGHT:	
SLEEP (hrs):	
CALORIES:	
TIME (minutes):	

Vitamin/ Supplements/ Meds

....

....

....

EXERCISES	SETS	Duration	Intensity	Cal/Burn

Blood Sugar Log	Before	After	Insulin
Breakfast			
Lunch			
Dinner			
Bedtime			

Note

____

____

Mood

Date _____ / _____ / _____   Day: _______   MO TU WE TH FR SA SU

Daily Food and Beverage Log

Food	BREAKFAST				
	Cals	Carbs	Fiber	Protein	Sugar
MEAL SUBTOTAL					

Food	LUNCH				
	Cals	Carbs	Fiber	Protein	Sugar
MEAL SUBTOTAL					

Food	DINNER				
	Cals	Carbs	Fiber	Protein	Sugar
MEAL SUBTOTAL					

Food	SNACKS				
	Cals	Carbs	Fiber	Protein	Sugar
MEAL SUBTOTAL					

DAILY GRAND TOTAL	Cals	Carbs	Fiber	Protein	Sugar	Met my goals today?	Yes	No

WORKOUT LOG

The exercise program and provides.

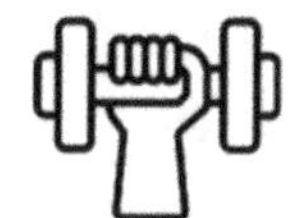

WEIGHT:	
SLEEP (hrs):	
CALORIES:	
TIME (minutes):	

EXERCISES	SETS	Duration	Intensity	Cal/Burn

Blood Sugar Log	Before	After	Insulin
Breakfast			
Lunch			
Dinner			
Bedtime			

Note

____

____

Mood

Date____/____/____   Day: ______   MO TU WE TH FR SA SU

Daily Food and Beverage Log

Food	BREAKFAST				
	Cals	Carbs	Fiber	Protein	Sugar
MEAL SUBTOTAL					

Food	LUNCH				
	Cals	Carbs	Fiber	Protein	Sugar
MEAL SUBTOTAL					

Food	DINNER				
	Cals	Carbs	Fiber	Protein	Sugar
MEAL SUBTOTAL					

Food	SNACKS				
	Cals	Carbs	Fiber	Protein	Sugar
MEAL SUBTOTAL					

DAILY GRAND TOTAL	Cals	Carbs	Fiber	Protein	Sugar	Met my goals today?	Yes	No

WORKOUT LOG

The exercise program and provides.

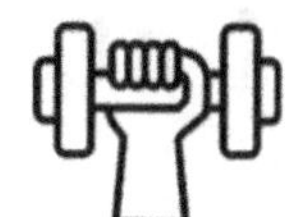

WEIGHT:	
SLEEP (hrs):	
CALORIES:	
TIME (minutes):	

EXERCISES	SETS	Duration	Intensity	Cal/Burn

Blood Sugar Log	Before	After	Insulin
Breakfast			
Lunch			
Dinner			
Bedtime			

Note

Mood

Daily Food and Beverage Log

Date_____/_____/_____   Day: ______   MO TU WE TH FR SA SU

Food	BREAKFAST				
	Cals	Carbs	Fiber	Protein	Sugar
MEAL SUBTOTAL					

Food	LUNCH				
	Cals	Carbs	Fiber	Protein	Sugar
MEAL SUBTOTAL					

Food	DINNER				
	Cals	Carbs	Fiber	Protein	Sugar
MEAL SUBTOTAL					

Food	SNACKS				
	Cals	Carbs	Fiber	Protein	Sugar
MEAL SUBTOTAL					

DAILY GRAND TOTAL	Cals	Carbs	Fiber	Protein	Sugar	Met my goals today?	Yes	No

WORKOUT LOG

The exercise program and provides.

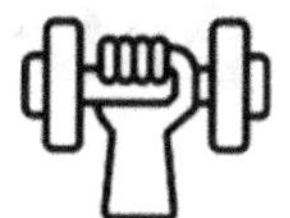

WEIGHT:	
SLEEP (hrs):	
CALORIES:	
TIME (minutes):	

EXERCISES	SETS	Duration	Intensity	Cal/Burn

Blood Sugar Log	Before	After	Insulin
Breakfast			
Lunch			
Dinner			
Bedtime			

Note

Mood

Date____/____/____ Day:______   MO TU WE TH FR SA SU

Daily Food and Beverage Log

Food	BREAKFAST				
	Cals	Carbs	Fiber	Protein	Sugar
MEAL SUBTOTAL					

Food	LUNCH				
	Cals	Carbs	Fiber	Protein	Sugar
MEAL SUBTOTAL					

Food	DINNER				
	Cals	Carbs	Fiber	Protein	Sugar
MEAL SUBTOTAL					

Food	SNACKS				
	Cals	Carbs	Fiber	Protein	Sugar
MEAL SUBTOTAL					

DAILY GRAND TOTAL	Cals	Carbs	Fiber	Protein	Sugar	Met my goals today?	Yes	No

WORKOUT LOG

The exercise program and provides.

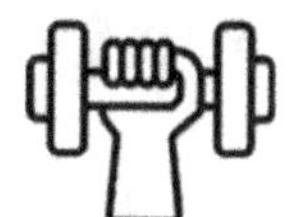

WEIGHT:	
SLEEP (hrs):	
CALORIES:	
TIME (minutes):	

EXERCISES	SETS	Duration	Intensity	Cal/Burn

Blood Sugar Log	Before	After	Insulin
Breakfast			
Lunch			
Dinner			
Bedtime			

Note

____

____

Mood

Date______ / ___ / ______   Day: ________   MO TU WE TH FR SA SU

Daily Food and Beverage Log

Food	BREAKFAST				
	Cals	Carbs	Fiber	Protein	Sugar
MEAL SUBTOTAL					

Food	LUNCH				
	Cals	Carbs	Fiber	Protein	Sugar
MEAL SUBTOTAL					

Food	DINNER				
	Cals	Carbs	Fiber	Protein	Sugar
MEAL SUBTOTAL					

Food	SNACKS				
	Cals	Carbs	Fiber	Protein	Sugar
MEAL SUBTOTAL					

DAILY GRAND TOTAL	Cals	Carbs	Fiber	Protein	Sugar	Met my goals today?	Yes	No

WORKOUT LOG

The exercise program and provides.

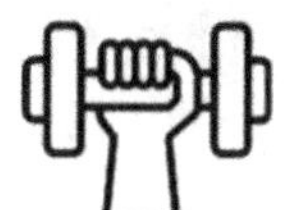

WEIGHT:	
SLEEP (hrs):	
CALORIES:	
TIME (minutes):	

Vitamin / Supplements / Meds

EXERCISES	SETS	Duration	Intensity	Cal/Burn

Blood Sugar Log	Before	After	Insulin
Breakfast			
Lunch			
Dinner			
Bedtime			

Note

Mood

Date____/____/____   Day: ______   MO TU WE TH FR SA SU

Daily Food and Beverage Log

Food	BREAKFAST				
	Cals	Carbs	Fiber	Protein	Sugar
MEAL SUBTOTAL					

Food	LUNCH				
	Cals	Carbs	Fiber	Protein	Sugar
MEAL SUBTOTAL					

Food	DINNER				
	Cals	Carbs	Fiber	Protein	Sugar
MEAL SUBTOTAL					

Food	SNACKS				
	Cals	Carbs	Fiber	Protein	Sugar
MEAL SUBTOTAL					

DAILY GRAND TOTAL	Cals	Carbs	Fiber	Protein	Sugar	Met my goals today?	Yes	No

WORKOUT LOG

The exercise program and provides.

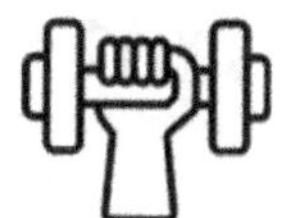

WEIGHT:	
SLEEP (hrs):	
CALORIES:	
TIME (minutes):	

EXERCISES	SETS	Duration	Intensity	Cal/Burn

Blood Sugar Log	Before	After	Insulin
Breakfast			
Lunch			
Dinner			
Bedtime			

Note

Mood

Date___/___/___   Day:______   MO TU WE TH FR SA SU

Daily Food and Beverage Log

Food	BREAKFAST				
	Cals	Carbs	Fiber	Protein	Sugar
MEAL SUBTOTAL					

Food	LUNCH				
	Cals	Carbs	Fiber	Protein	Sugar
MEAL SUBTOTAL					

Food	DINNER				
	Cals	Carbs	Fiber	Protein	Sugar
MEAL SUBTOTAL					

Food	SNACKS				
	Cals	Carbs	Fiber	Protein	Sugar
MEAL SUBTOTAL					

DAILY GRAND TOTAL	Cals	Carbs	Fiber	Protein	Sugar	Met my goals today?	Yes	No

WORKOUT LOG

The exercise program and provides.

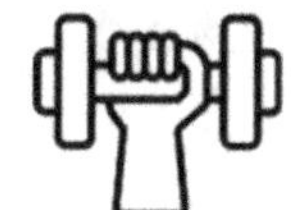

WEIGHT:	
SLEEP (hrs):	
CALORIES:	
TIME (minutes):	

Vitamin/ Supplements/ Meds

....

....

....

EXERCISES	SETS	Duration	Intensity	Cal/Burn

Blood Sugar Log	Before	After	Insulin
Breakfast			
Lunch			
Dinner			
Bedtime			

Note

____

____

Mood

Date______/______/______   Day:_______   MO TU WE TH FR SA SU

Daily Food and Beverage Log

Food	BREAKFAST				
	Cals	Carbs	Fiber	Protein	Sugar
MEAL SUBTOTAL					

Food	LUNCH				
	Cals	Carbs	Fiber	Protein	Sugar
MEAL SUBTOTAL					

Food	DINNER				
	Cals	Carbs	Fiber	Protein	Sugar
MEAL SUBTOTAL					

Food	SNACKS				
	Cals	Carbs	Fiber	Protein	Sugar
MEAL SUBTOTAL					

DAILY GRAND TOTAL	Cals	Carbs	Fiber	Protein	Sugar	Met my goals today?	Yes	No

WORKOUT LOG

The exercise program and provides.

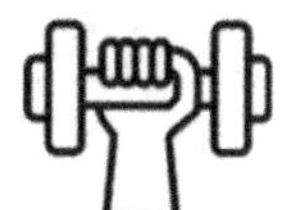

WEIGHT:	
SLEEP (hrs):	
CALORIES:	
TIME (minutes):	

EXERCISES	SETS	Duration	Intensity	Cal/Burn

Blood Sugar Log	Before	After	Insulin
Breakfast			
Lunch			
Dinner			
Bedtime			

Note

Mood

Daily Food and Beverage Log

Date_____/_____/_____   Day:_______   MO TU WE TH FR SA SU

Food	BREAKFAST				
	Cals	Carbs	Fiber	Protein	Sugar
MEAL SUBTOTAL					

Food	LUNCH				
	Cals	Carbs	Fiber	Protein	Sugar
MEAL SUBTOTAL					

Food	DINNER				
	Cals	Carbs	Fiber	Protein	Sugar
MEAL SUBTOTAL					

Food	SNACKS				
	Cals	Carbs	Fiber	Protein	Sugar
MEAL SUBTOTAL					

DAILY GRAND TOTAL	Cals	Carbs	Fiber	Protein	Sugar	Met my goals today?	Yes	No

WORKOUT LOG

The exercise program and provides.

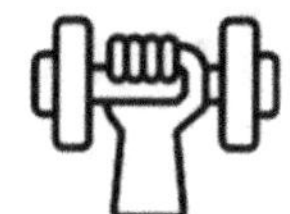

WEIGHT:	
SLEEP (hrs):	
CALORIES:	
TIME (minutes):	

EXERCISES	SETS	Duration	Intensity	Cal/Burn

Blood Sugar Log	Before	After	Insulin
Breakfast			
Lunch			
Dinner			
Bedtime			

Note

Mood

Daily Food and Beverage Log

Date ___/___/___ Day: ______ MO TU WE TH FR SA SU

Food	BREAKFAST				
	Cals	Carbs	Fiber	Protein	Sugar
MEAL SUBTOTAL					

Food	LUNCH				
	Cals	Carbs	Fiber	Protein	Sugar
MEAL SUBTOTAL					

Food	DINNER				
	Cals	Carbs	Fiber	Protein	Sugar
MEAL SUBTOTAL					

Food	SNACKS				
	Cals	Carbs	Fiber	Protein	Sugar
MEAL SUBTOTAL					

DAILY GRAND TOTAL	Cals	Carbs	Fiber	Protein	Sugar	Met my goals today?	Yes	No

WORKOUT LOG

The exercise program and provides.

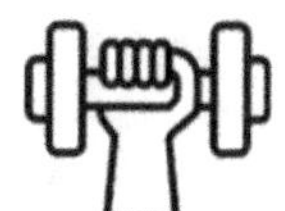

WEIGHT:	
SLEEP (hrs):	
CALORIES:	
TIME (minutes):	

Vitamin / Supplements / Meds

....

....

EXERCISES	SETS	Duration	Intensity	Cal/Burn

Blood Sugar Log	Before	After	Insulin
Breakfast			
Lunch			
Dinner			
Bedtime			

Note

____

____

Mood

Date___/___/___   Day:______   MO TU WE TH FR SA SU

Daily Food and Beverage Log

Food	BREAKFAST				
	Cals	Carbs	Fiber	Protein	Sugar
MEAL SUBTOTAL					

Food	LUNCH				
	Cals	Carbs	Fiber	Protein	Sugar
MEAL SUBTOTAL					

Food	DINNER				
	Cals	Carbs	Fiber	Protein	Sugar
MEAL SUBTOTAL					

Food	SNACKS				
	Cals	Carbs	Fiber	Protein	Sugar
MEAL SUBTOTAL					

DAILY GRAND TOTAL	Cals	Carbs	Fiber	Protein	Sugar	Met my goals today?	Yes	No

WORKOUT LOG

The exercise program and provides.

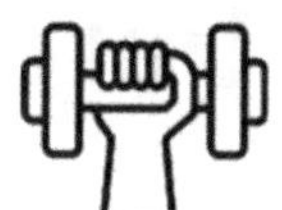

WEIGHT:	
SLEEP (hrs):	
CALORIES:	
TIME (minutes):	

Vitamin / Supplements / Meds

EXERCISES	SETS	Duration	Intensity	Cal/Burn

Blood Sugar Log	Before	After	Insulin
Breakfast			
Lunch			
Dinner			
Bedtime			

Note

Mood

Date____/____/____   Day: ______   MO TU WE TH FR SA SU

Daily Food and Beverage Log

Food	BREAKFAST				
	Cals	Carbs	Fiber	Protein	Sugar
MEAL SUBTOTAL					

Food	LUNCH				
	Cals	Carbs	Fiber	Protein	Sugar
MEAL SUBTOTAL					

Food	DINNER				
	Cals	Carbs	Fiber	Protein	Sugar
MEAL SUBTOTAL					

Food	SNACKS				
	Cals	Carbs	Fiber	Protein	Sugar
MEAL SUBTOTAL					

DAILY GRAND TOTAL	Cals	Carbs	Fiber	Protein	Sugar	Met my goals today?	Yes	No

WORKOUT LOG

The exercise program and provides.

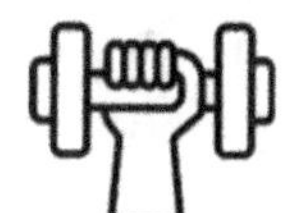

WEIGHT:	
SLEEP (hrs):	
CALORIES:	
TIME (minutes):	

EXERCISES	SETS	Duration	Intensity	Cal/Burn

Blood Sugar Log	Before	After	Insulin
Breakfast			
Lunch			
Dinner			
Bedtime			

Note

____

____

Mood

Date____/____/____   Day:______   MO TU WE TH FR SA SU

Daily Food and Beverage Log

Food	BREAKFAST				
	Cals	Carbs	Fiber	Protein	Sugar
MEAL SUBTOTAL					

Food	LUNCH				
	Cals	Carbs	Fiber	Protein	Sugar
MEAL SUBTOTAL					

Food	DINNER				
	Cals	Carbs	Fiber	Protein	Sugar
MEAL SUBTOTAL					

Food	SNACKS				
	Cals	Carbs	Fiber	Protein	Sugar
MEAL SUBTOTAL					

DAILY GRAND TOTAL	Cals	Carbs	Fiber	Protein	Sugar	Met my goals today?	Yes	No

WORKOUT LOG

The exercise program and provides.

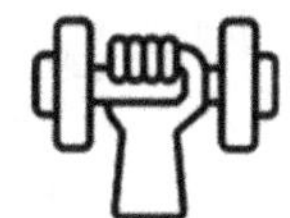

WEIGHT:	
SLEEP (hrs):	
CALORIES:	
TIME (minutes):	

EXERCISES	SETS	Duration	Intensity	Cal/Burn

Blood Sugar Log	Before	After	Insulin
Breakfast			
Lunch			
Dinner			
Bedtime			

Note

Mood

Date____/____/____ Day:______ MO TU WE TH FR SA SU

Daily Food and Beverage Log

Food	BREAKFAST				
	Cals	Carbs	Fiber	Protein	Sugar
MEAL SUBTOTAL					

Food	LUNCH				
	Cals	Carbs	Fiber	Protein	Sugar
MEAL SUBTOTAL					

Food	DINNER				
	Cals	Carbs	Fiber	Protein	Sugar
MEAL SUBTOTAL					

Food	SNACKS				
	Cals	Carbs	Fiber	Protein	Sugar
MEAL SUBTOTAL					

DAILY GRAND TOTAL	Cals	Carbs	Fiber	Protein	Sugar	Met my goals today?	Yes	No

WORKOUT LOG

The exercise program and provides.

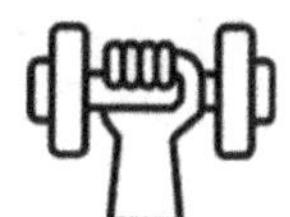

WEIGHT:	
SLEEP (hrs):	
CALORIES:	
TIME (minutes):	

EXERCISES	SETS	Duration	Intensity	Cal/Burn

Blood Sugar Log	Before	After	Insulin
Breakfast			
Lunch			
Dinner			
Bedtime			

Note

Mood

Date_____ / _____ / _____   Day: _______   MO TU WE TH FR SA SU

Daily Food and Beverage Log

Food	BREAKFAST				
	Cals	Carbs	Fiber	Protein	Sugar
MEAL SUBTOTAL					

Food	LUNCH				
	Cals	Carbs	Fiber	Protein	Sugar
MEAL SUBTOTAL					

Food	DINNER				
	Cals	Carbs	Fiber	Protein	Sugar
MEAL SUBTOTAL					

Food	SNACKS				
	Cals	Carbs	Fiber	Protein	Sugar
MEAL SUBTOTAL					

DAILY GRAND TOTAL	Cals	Carbs	Fiber	Protein	Sugar	Met my goals today?	Yes	No

WORKOUT LOG

The exercise program and provides.

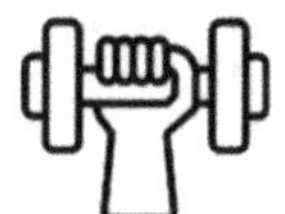

WEIGHT:	
SLEEP (hrs):	
CALORIES:	
TIME (minutes):	

EXERCISES	SETS	Duration	Intensity	Cal/Burn

Blood Sugar Log	Before	After	Insulin
Breakfast			
Lunch			
Dinner			
Bedtime			

Note

Mood

Date_____/_____/_____   Day:_______   MO TU WE TH FR SA SU

Daily Food and Beverage Log

Food	BREAKFAST				
	Cals	Carbs	Fiber	Protein	Sugar
MEAL SUBTOTAL					

Food	LUNCH				
	Cals	Carbs	Fiber	Protein	Sugar
MEAL SUBTOTAL					

Food	DINNER				
	Cals	Carbs	Fiber	Protein	Sugar
MEAL SUBTOTAL					

Food	SNACKS				
	Cals	Carbs	Fiber	Protein	Sugar
MEAL SUBTOTAL					

DAILY GRAND TOTAL	Cals	Carbs	Fiber	Protein	Sugar	Met my goals today?	Yes	No

WORKOUT LOG

The exercise program and provides.

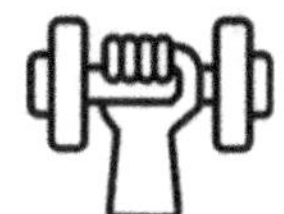

WEIGHT:	
SLEEP (hrs):	
CALORIES:	
TIME (minutes):	

EXERCISES	SETS	Duration	Intensity	Cal/Burn

Blood Sugar Log	Before	After	Insulin
Breakfast			
Lunch			
Dinner			
Bedtime			

Note

Mood

Date____/____/____   Day: ______   MO TU WE TH FR SA SU

Daily Food and Beverage Log

Food	BREAKFAST				
	Cals	Carbs	Fiber	Protein	Sugar
MEAL SUBTOTAL					

Food	LUNCH				
	Cals	Carbs	Fiber	Protein	Sugar
MEAL SUBTOTAL					

Food	DINNER				
	Cals	Carbs	Fiber	Protein	Sugar
MEAL SUBTOTAL					

Food	SNACKS				
	Cals	Carbs	Fiber	Protein	Sugar
MEAL SUBTOTAL					

DAILY GRAND TOTAL	Cals	Carbs	Fiber	Protein	Sugar	Met my goals today?	Yes	No

WORKOUT LOG

The exercise program and provides.

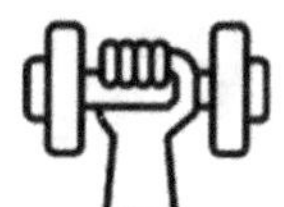

WEIGHT:	
SLEEP (hrs):	
CALORIES:	
TIME (minutes):	

EXERCISES	SETS	Duration	Intensity	Cal/Burn

Blood Sugar Log	Before	After	Insulin
Breakfast			
Lunch			
Dinner			
Bedtime			

Note

Mood

Date______/______/______   Day: ______   MO TU WE TH FR SA SU

Daily Food and Beverage Log

Food	BREAKFAST				
	Cals	Carbs	Fiber	Protein	Sugar
MEAL SUBTOTAL					

Food	LUNCH				
	Cals	Carbs	Fiber	Protein	Sugar
MEAL SUBTOTAL					

Food	DINNER				
	Cals	Carbs	Fiber	Protein	Sugar
MEAL SUBTOTAL					

Food	SNACKS				
	Cals	Carbs	Fiber	Protein	Sugar
MEAL SUBTOTAL					

DAILY GRAND TOTAL	Cals	Carbs	Fiber	Protein	Sugar	Met my goals today?	Yes	No

WORKOUT LOG

The exercise program and provides.

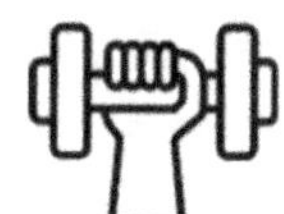

WEIGHT:	
SLEEP (hrs):	
CALORIES:	
TIME (minutes):	

EXERCISES	SETS	Duration	Intensity	Cal/Burn

Blood Sugar Log	Before	After	Insulin
Breakfast			
Lunch			
Dinner			
Bedtime			

Note

Mood

Date____/____/____ Day:______ MO TU WE TH FR SA SU

Daily Food and Beverage Log

Food	BREAKFAST				
	Cals	Carbs	Fiber	Protein	Sugar
MEAL SUBTOTAL					

Food	LUNCH				
	Cals	Carbs	Fiber	Protein	Sugar
MEAL SUBTOTAL					

Food	DINNER				
	Cals	Carbs	Fiber	Protein	Sugar
MEAL SUBTOTAL					

Food	SNACKS				
	Cals	Carbs	Fiber	Protein	Sugar
MEAL SUBTOTAL					

DAILY GRAND TOTAL	Cals	Carbs	Fiber	Protein	Sugar	Met my goals today?	Yes	No

WORKOUT LOG

The exercise program and provides.

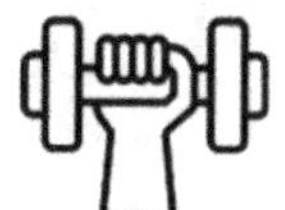

WEIGHT:	
SLEEP (hrs):	
CALORIES:	
TIME (minutes):	

EXERCISES	SETS	Duration	Intensity	Cal/Burn

Blood Sugar Log	Before	After	Insulin
Breakfast			
Lunch			
Dinner			
Bedtime			

Note

Mood

Daily Food and Beverage Log

Date____/____/____   Day:______   MO TU WE TH FR SA SU

Food	BREAKFAST				
	Cals	Carbs	Fiber	Protein	Sugar
MEAL SUBTOTAL					

Food	LUNCH				
	Cals	Carbs	Fiber	Protein	Sugar
MEAL SUBTOTAL					

Food	DINNER				
	Cals	Carbs	Fiber	Protein	Sugar
MEAL SUBTOTAL					

Food	SNACKS				
	Cals	Carbs	Fiber	Protein	Sugar
MEAL SUBTOTAL					

DAILY GRAND TOTAL	Cals	Carbs	Fiber	Protein	Sugar	Met my goals today?	Yes	No

WORKOUT LOG

The exercise program and provides.

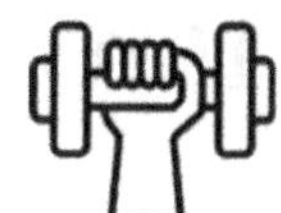

WEIGHT:	
SLEEP (hrs):	
CALORIES:	
TIME (minutes):	

EXERCISES	SETS	Duration	Intensity	Cal/Burn

Blood Sugar Log	Before	After	Insulin
Breakfast			
Lunch			
Dinner			
Bedtime			

Note

Mood

Date___/___/___   Day: ______   MO TU WE TH FR SA SU

Daily Food and Beverage Log

Food	BREAKFAST				
	Cals	Carbs	Fiber	Protein	Sugar
MEAL SUBTOTAL					

Food	LUNCH				
	Cals	Carbs	Fiber	Protein	Sugar
MEAL SUBTOTAL					

Food	DINNER				
	Cals	Carbs	Fiber	Protein	Sugar
MEAL SUBTOTAL					

Food	SNACKS				
	Cals	Carbs	Fiber	Protein	Sugar
MEAL SUBTOTAL					

DAILY GRAND TOTAL	Cals	Carbs	Fiber	Protein	Sugar	Met my goals today?	Yes	No

WORKOUT LOG

The exercise program and provides.

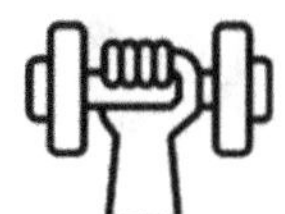

WEIGHT:	
SLEEP (hrs):	
CALORIES:	
TIME (minutes):	

Vitamin/ Supplements/ Meds

EXERCISES	SETS	Duration	Intensity	Cal/Burn

Blood Sugar Log	Before	After	Insulin
Breakfast			
Lunch			
Dinner			
Bedtime			

Note

Mood

Daily Food and Beverage Log

Date______/______/______   Day: ______   MO TU WE TH FR SA SU

Food	BREAKFAST				
	Cals	Carbs	Fiber	Protein	Sugar
MEAL SUBTOTAL					

Food	LUNCH				
	Cals	Carbs	Fiber	Protein	Sugar
MEAL SUBTOTAL					

Food	DINNER				
	Cals	Carbs	Fiber	Protein	Sugar
MEAL SUBTOTAL					

Food	SNACKS				
	Cals	Carbs	Fiber	Protein	Sugar
MEAL SUBTOTAL					

DAILY GRAND TOTAL	Cals	Carbs	Fiber	Protein	Sugar	Met my goals today?	Yes	No

WORKOUT LOG

The exercise program and provides.

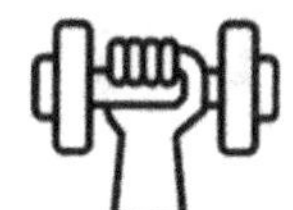

WEIGHT:	
SLEEP (hrs):	
CALORIES:	
TIME (minutes):	

Vitamin/ Supplements/ Meds

....

....

....

EXERCISES	SETS	Duration	Intensity	Cal/Burn

Blood Sugar Log	Before	After	Insulin
Breakfast			
Lunch			
Dinner			
Bedtime			

Note

____

____

Mood

Date_____/_____/_____   Day:_______   MO TU WE TH FR SA SU

Daily Food and Beverage Log

Food	BREAKFAST				
	Cals	Carbs	Fiber	Protein	Sugar
MEAL SUBTOTAL					

Food	LUNCH				
	Cals	Carbs	Fiber	Protein	Sugar
MEAL SUBTOTAL					

Food	DINNER				
	Cals	Carbs	Fiber	Protein	Sugar
MEAL SUBTOTAL					

Food	SNACKS				
	Cals	Carbs	Fiber	Protein	Sugar
MEAL SUBTOTAL					

DAILY GRAND TOTAL	Cals	Carbs	Fiber	Protein	Sugar	Met my goals today?	Yes	No

WORKOUT LOG

The exercise program and provides.

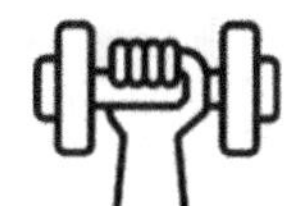

WEIGHT:	
SLEEP (hrs):	
CALORIES:	
TIME (minutes):	

EXERCISES	SETS	Duration	Intensity	Cal/Burn

Blood Sugar Log	Before	After	Insulin
Breakfast			
Lunch			
Dinner			
Bedtime			

Note

Mood

Date_____ / _____ / _____   Day: _______   MO TU WE TH FR SA SU

Daily Food and Beverage Log

Food	BREAKFAST				
	Cals	Carbs	Fiber	Protein	Sugar
MEAL SUBTOTAL					

Food	LUNCH				
	Cals	Carbs	Fiber	Protein	Sugar
MEAL SUBTOTAL					

Food	DINNER				
	Cals	Carbs	Fiber	Protein	Sugar
MEAL SUBTOTAL					

Food	SNACKS				
	Cals	Carbs	Fiber	Protein	Sugar
MEAL SUBTOTAL					

DAILY GRAND TOTAL	Cals	Carbs	Fiber	Protein	Sugar	Met my goals today?	Yes	No

WORKOUT LOG

The exercise program and provides.

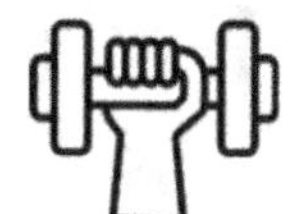

WEIGHT:	
SLEEP (hrs):	
CALORIES:	
TIME (minutes):	

EXERCISES	SETS	Duration	Intensity	Cal/Burn

Blood Sugar Log	Before	After	Insulin
Breakfast			
Lunch			
Dinner			
Bedtime			

Note

Mood

Date______/______/______   Day: ________   MO TU WE TH FR SA SU

Daily Food and Beverage Log

Food	BREAKFAST				
	Cals	Carbs	Fiber	Protein	Sugar
MEAL SUBTOTAL					

Food	LUNCH				
	Cals	Carbs	Fiber	Protein	Sugar
MEAL SUBTOTAL					

Food	DINNER				
	Cals	Carbs	Fiber	Protein	Sugar
MEAL SUBTOTAL					

Food	SNACKS				
	Cals	Carbs	Fiber	Protein	Sugar
MEAL SUBTOTAL					

DAILY GRAND TOTAL	Cals	Carbs	Fiber	Protein	Sugar	Met my goals today?	Yes	No

WORKOUT LOG

The exercise program and provides.

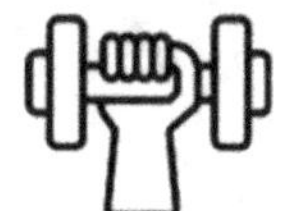

WEIGHT:	
SLEEP (hrs):	
CALORIES:	
TIME (minutes):	

Vitamin/Supplements/Meds

EXERCISES	SETS	Duration	Intensity	Cal/Burn

Blood Sugar Log	Before	After	Insulin
Breakfast			
Lunch			
Dinner			
Bedtime			

Note

Mood

Date_____/_____/_____   Day: ______   MO TU WE TH FR SA SU

Daily Food and Beverage Log

Food	BREAKFAST				
	Cals	Carbs	Fiber	Protein	Sugar
MEAL SUBTOTAL					

Food	LUNCH				
	Cals	Carbs	Fiber	Protein	Sugar
MEAL SUBTOTAL					

Food	DINNER				
	Cals	Carbs	Fiber	Protein	Sugar
MEAL SUBTOTAL					

Food	SNACKS				
	Cals	Carbs	Fiber	Protein	Sugar
MEAL SUBTOTAL					

DAILY GRAND TOTAL	Cals	Carbs	Fiber	Protein	Sugar	Met my goals today?	Yes	No

WORKOUT LOG

The exercise program and provides.

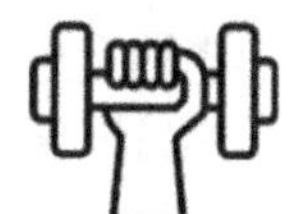

WEIGHT:	
SLEEP (hrs):	
CALORIES:	
TIME (minutes):	

EXERCISES	SETS	Duration	Intensity	Cal/Burn

Blood Sugar Log	Before	After	Insulin
Breakfast			
Lunch			
Dinner			
Bedtime			

Note

Mood

Date____/____/____ Day: ______ MO TU WE TH FR SA SU

Daily Food and Beverage Log

Food	BREAKFAST				
	Cals	Carbs	Fiber	Protein	Sugar
MEAL SUBTOTAL					

Food	LUNCH				
	Cals	Carbs	Fiber	Protein	Sugar
MEAL SUBTOTAL					

Food	DINNER				
	Cals	Carbs	Fiber	Protein	Sugar
MEAL SUBTOTAL					

Food	SNACKS				
	Cals	Carbs	Fiber	Protein	Sugar
MEAL SUBTOTAL					

DAILY GRAND TOTAL	Cals	Carbs	Fiber	Protein	Sugar	Met my goals today?	Yes	No

WORKOUT LOG

The exercise program and provides.

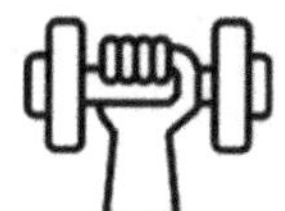

WEIGHT:	
SLEEP (hrs):	
CALORIES:	
TIME (minutes):	

EXERCISES	SETS	Duration	Intensity	Cal/Burn

Blood Sugar Log	Before	After	Insulin
Breakfast			
Lunch			
Dinner			
Bedtime			

Note

Mood

Date____/____/____ Day:______ MO TU WE TH FR SA SU

Daily Food and Beverage Log

Food	BREAKFAST				
	Cals	Carbs	Fiber	Protein	Sugar
MEAL SUBTOTAL					

Food	LUNCH				
	Cals	Carbs	Fiber	Protein	Sugar
MEAL SUBTOTAL					

Food	DINNER				
	Cals	Carbs	Fiber	Protein	Sugar
MEAL SUBTOTAL					

Food	SNACKS				
	Cals	Carbs	Fiber	Protein	Sugar
MEAL SUBTOTAL					

DAILY GRAND TOTAL	Cals	Carbs	Fiber	Protein	Sugar	Met my goals today?	Yes	No

WORKOUT LOG

The exercise program and provides.

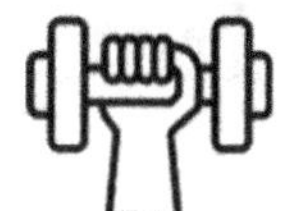

WEIGHT:	
SLEEP (hrs):	
CALORIES:	
TIME (minutes):	

Vitamin / Supplements / Meds

EXERCISES	SETS	Duration	Intensity	Cal/Burn

Blood Sugar Log	Before	After	Insulin
Breakfast			
Lunch			
Dinner			
Bedtime			

Note

Mood

Date____/____/____   Day:______   MO TU WE TH FR SA SU

Daily Food and Beverage Log

Food	BREAKFAST				
	Cals	Carbs	Fiber	Protein	Sugar
MEAL SUBTOTAL					

Food	LUNCH				
	Cals	Carbs	Fiber	Protein	Sugar
MEAL SUBTOTAL					

Food	DINNER				
	Cals	Carbs	Fiber	Protein	Sugar
MEAL SUBTOTAL					

Food	SNACKS				
	Cals	Carbs	Fiber	Protein	Sugar
MEAL SUBTOTAL					

DAILY GRAND TOTAL	Cals	Carbs	Fiber	Protein	Sugar	Met my goals today?	Yes	No

WORKOUT LOG

The exercise program and provides.

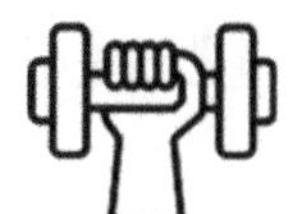

WEIGHT:	
SLEEP (hrs):	
CALORIES:	
TIME (minutes):	

Vitamin/ Supplements/ Meds

....

....

....

EXERCISES	SETS	Duration	Intensity	Cal/Burn

Blood Sugar Log	Before	After	Insulin
Breakfast			
Lunch			
Dinner			
Bedtime			

Note

____

____

Mood

Date_____/_____/_____ Day:_______ MO TU WE TH FR SA SU

Daily Food and Beverage Log

Food	BREAKFAST				
	Cals	Carbs	Fiber	Protein	Sugar
MEAL SUBTOTAL					

Food	LUNCH				
	Cals	Carbs	Fiber	Protein	Sugar
MEAL SUBTOTAL					

Food	DINNER				
	Cals	Carbs	Fiber	Protein	Sugar
MEAL SUBTOTAL					

Food	SNACKS				
	Cals	Carbs	Fiber	Protein	Sugar
MEAL SUBTOTAL					

DAILY GRAND TOTAL	Cals	Carbs	Fiber	Protein	Sugar	Met my goals today?	Yes	No

WORKOUT LOG

The exercise program and provides.

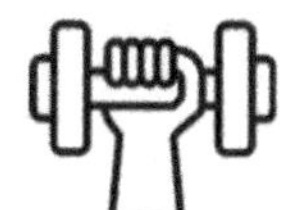

WEIGHT:	
SLEEP (hrs):	
CALORIES:	
TIME (minutes):	

EXERCISES	SETS	Duration	Intensity	Cal/Burn

Blood Sugar Log	Before	After	Insulin
Breakfast			
Lunch			
Dinner			
Bedtime			

Note

Mood

Date____/____/____   Day: ______   MO TU WE TH FR SA SU

Daily Food and Beverage Log

Food	BREAKFAST				
	Cals	Carbs	Fiber	Protein	Sugar
MEAL SUBTOTAL					

Food	LUNCH				
	Cals	Carbs	Fiber	Protein	Sugar
MEAL SUBTOTAL					

Food	DINNER				
	Cals	Carbs	Fiber	Protein	Sugar
MEAL SUBTOTAL					

Food	SNACKS				
	Cals	Carbs	Fiber	Protein	Sugar
MEAL SUBTOTAL					

DAILY GRAND TOTAL	Cals	Carbs	Fiber	Protein	Sugar	Met my goals today?	Yes	No

WORKOUT LOG

The exercise program and provides.

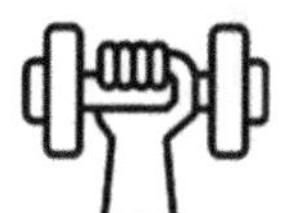

WEIGHT:	
SLEEP (hrs):	
CALORIES:	
TIME (minutes):	

EXERCISES	SETS	Duration	Intensity	Cal/Burn

Blood Sugar Log	Before	After	Insulin
Breakfast			
Lunch			
Dinner			
Bedtime			

Note

____

____

Mood

Daily Food and Beverage Log

Date______/______/______   Day: ______   MO TU WE TH FR SA SU

Food	BREAKFAST				
	Cals	Carbs	Fiber	Protein	Sugar
MEAL SUBTOTAL					

Food	LUNCH				
	Cals	Carbs	Fiber	Protein	Sugar
MEAL SUBTOTAL					

Food	DINNER				
	Cals	Carbs	Fiber	Protein	Sugar
MEAL SUBTOTAL					

Food	SNACKS				
	Cals	Carbs	Fiber	Protein	Sugar
MEAL SUBTOTAL					

DAILY GRAND TOTAL	Cals	Carbs	Fiber	Protein	Sugar	Met my goals today?	Yes	No

WORKOUT LOG

The exercise program and provides.

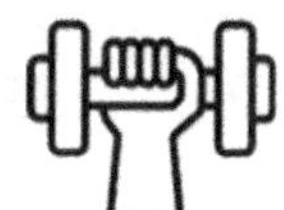

WEIGHT:	
SLEEP (hrs):	
CALORIES:	
TIME (minutes):	

EXERCISES	SETS	Duration	Intensity	Cal/Burn

Blood Sugar Log	Before	After	Insulin
Breakfast			
Lunch			
Dinner			
Bedtime			

Note

Mood

Date___/___/___   Day: ______   MO TU WE TH FR SA SU

Daily Food and Beverage Log

Food	BREAKFAST				
	Cals	Carbs	Fiber	Protein	Sugar
MEAL SUBTOTAL					

Food	LUNCH				
	Cals	Carbs	Fiber	Protein	Sugar
MEAL SUBTOTAL					

Food	DINNER				
	Cals	Carbs	Fiber	Protein	Sugar
MEAL SUBTOTAL					

Food	SNACKS				
	Cals	Carbs	Fiber	Protein	Sugar
MEAL SUBTOTAL					

DAILY GRAND TOTAL	Cals	Carbs	Fiber	Protein	Sugar	Met my goals today?	Yes	No

WORKOUT LOG

The exercise program and provides.

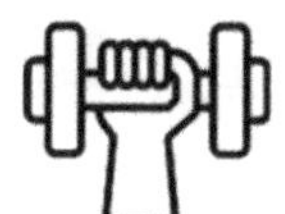

WEIGHT:	
SLEEP (hrs):	
CALORIES:	
TIME (minutes):	

EXERCISES	SETS	Duration	Intensity	Cal/Burn

Blood Sugar Log	Before	After	Insulin
Breakfast			
Lunch			
Dinner			
Bedtime			

Note

____

Mood

Date____/____/____   Day:______   MO TU WE TH FR SA SU

Daily Food and Beverage Log

Food	BREAKFAST				
	Cals	Carbs	Fiber	Protein	Sugar
MEAL SUBTOTAL					

Food	LUNCH				
	Cals	Carbs	Fiber	Protein	Sugar
MEAL SUBTOTAL					

Food	DINNER				
	Cals	Carbs	Fiber	Protein	Sugar
MEAL SUBTOTAL					

Food	SNACKS				
	Cals	Carbs	Fiber	Protein	Sugar
MEAL SUBTOTAL					

DAILY GRAND TOTAL	Cals	Carbs	Fiber	Protein	Sugar	Met my goals today?	Yes	No

WORKOUT LOG

The exercise program and provides.

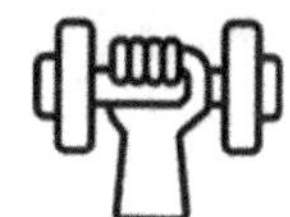

WEIGHT:	
SLEEP (hrs):	
CALORIES:	
TIME (minutes):	

EXERCISES	SETS	Duration	Intensity	Cal/Burn

Blood Sugar Log	Before	After	Insulin
Breakfast			
Lunch			
Dinner			
Bedtime			

Note

Mood

Date____/____/____   Day: ______   MO TU WE TH FR SA SU

Daily Food and Beverage Log

Food	BREAKFAST				
	Cals	Carbs	Fiber	Protein	Sugar
MEAL SUBTOTAL					

Food	LUNCH				
	Cals	Carbs	Fiber	Protein	Sugar
MEAL SUBTOTAL					

Food	DINNER				
	Cals	Carbs	Fiber	Protein	Sugar
MEAL SUBTOTAL					

Food	SNACKS				
	Cals	Carbs	Fiber	Protein	Sugar
MEAL SUBTOTAL					

DAILY GRAND TOTAL	Cals	Carbs	Fiber	Protein	Sugar	Met my goals today?	Yes	No

WORKOUT LOG

The exercise program and provides.

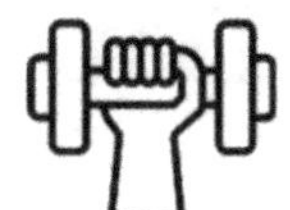

WEIGHT:	
SLEEP (hrs):	
CALORIES:	
TIME (minutes):	

EXERCISES	SETS	Duration	Intensity	Cal/Burn

Blood Sugar Log	Before	After	Insulin
Breakfast			
Lunch			
Dinner			
Bedtime			

Note

Mood

Date_____/_____/_____   Day:_______   MO TU WE TH FR SA SU

Daily Food and Beverage Log

Food	BREAKFAST				
	Cals	Carbs	Fiber	Protein	Sugar
MEAL SUBTOTAL					

Food	LUNCH				
	Cals	Carbs	Fiber	Protein	Sugar
MEAL SUBTOTAL					

Food	DINNER				
	Cals	Carbs	Fiber	Protein	Sugar
MEAL SUBTOTAL					

Food	SNACKS				
	Cals	Carbs	Fiber	Protein	Sugar
MEAL SUBTOTAL					

DAILY GRAND TOTAL	Cals	Carbs	Fiber	Protein	Sugar	Met my goals today?	Yes	No

WORKOUT LOG

The exercise program and provides.

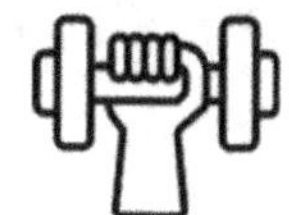

WEIGHT:	
SLEEP (hrs):	
CALORIES:	
TIME (minutes):	

EXERCISES	SETS	Duration	Intensity	Cal/Burn

Blood Sugar Log	Before	After	Insulin
Breakfast			
Lunch			
Dinner			
Bedtime			

Note

Mood

Date____/____/____   Day:______   MO TU WE TH FR SA SU

Daily Food and Beverage Log

Food	BREAKFAST				
	Cals	Carbs	Fiber	Protein	Sugar
MEAL SUBTOTAL					

Food	LUNCH				
	Cals	Carbs	Fiber	Protein	Sugar
MEAL SUBTOTAL					

Food	DINNER				
	Cals	Carbs	Fiber	Protein	Sugar
MEAL SUBTOTAL					

Food	SNACKS				
	Cals	Carbs	Fiber	Protein	Sugar
MEAL SUBTOTAL					

DAILY GRAND TOTAL	Cals	Carbs	Fiber	Protein	Sugar	Met my goals today?	Yes	No

WORKOUT LOG

The exercise program and provides.

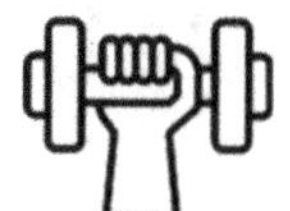

WEIGHT:	
SLEEP (hrs):	
CALORIES:	
TIME (minutes):	

EXERCISES	SETS	Duration	Intensity	Cal/Burn

Blood Sugar Log	Before	After	Insulin
Breakfast			
Lunch			
Dinner			
Bedtime			

Note

Mood

Date_____/_____/_____   Day: _______   MO TU WE TH FR SA SU

Daily Food and Beverage Log

Food	BREAKFAST				
	Cals	Carbs	Fiber	Protein	Sugar
MEAL SUBTOTAL					

Food	LUNCH				
	Cals	Carbs	Fiber	Protein	Sugar
MEAL SUBTOTAL					

Food	DINNER				
	Cals	Carbs	Fiber	Protein	Sugar
MEAL SUBTOTAL					

Food	SNACKS				
	Cals	Carbs	Fiber	Protein	Sugar
MEAL SUBTOTAL					

DAILY GRAND TOTAL	Cals	Carbs	Fiber	Protein	Sugar	Met my goals today?	Yes	No

WORKOUT LOG

The exercise program and provides.

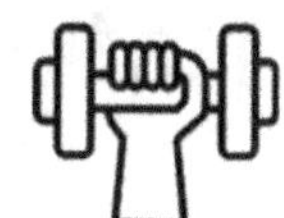

WEIGHT:	
SLEEP (hrs):	
CALORIES:	
TIME (minutes):	

EXERCISES	SETS	Duration	Intensity	Cal/Burn

Blood Sugar Log	Before	After	Insulin
Breakfast			
Lunch			
Dinner			
Bedtime			

Note

____

____

Mood

Date_____ / _____ / _____   Day: _______   MO TU WE TH FR SA SU

Daily Food and Beverage Log

Food	BREAKFAST				
	Cals	Carbs	Fiber	Protein	Sugar
MEAL SUBTOTAL					

Food	LUNCH				
	Cals	Carbs	Fiber	Protein	Sugar
MEAL SUBTOTAL					

Food	DINNER				
	Cals	Carbs	Fiber	Protein	Sugar
MEAL SUBTOTAL					

Food	SNACKS				
	Cals	Carbs	Fiber	Protein	Sugar
MEAL SUBTOTAL					

DAILY GRAND TOTAL	Cals	Carbs	Fiber	Protein	Sugar	Met my goals today?	Yes	No

WORKOUT LOG

The exercise program and provides.

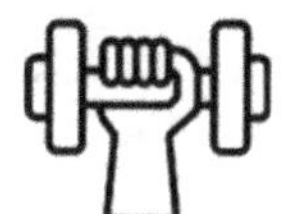

WEIGHT:	
SLEEP (hrs):	
CALORIES:	
TIME (minutes):	

EXERCISES	SETS	Duration	Intensity	Cal/Burn

Blood Sugar Log	Before	After	Insulin
Breakfast			
Lunch			
Dinner			
Bedtime			

Note

Mood

Date_____/_____/_____   Day:_______   MO TU WE TH FR SA SU

Daily Food and Beverage Log

Food	BREAKFAST				
	Cals	Carbs	Fiber	Protein	Sugar
MEAL SUBTOTAL					

Food	LUNCH				
	Cals	Carbs	Fiber	Protein	Sugar
MEAL SUBTOTAL					

Food	DINNER				
	Cals	Carbs	Fiber	Protein	Sugar
MEAL SUBTOTAL					

Food	SNACKS				
	Cals	Carbs	Fiber	Protein	Sugar
MEAL SUBTOTAL					

DAILY GRAND TOTAL	Cals	Carbs	Fiber	Protein	Sugar	Met my goals today?	Yes	No

WORKOUT LOG

The exercise program and provides.

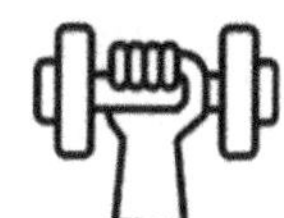

WEIGHT:	
SLEEP (hrs):	
CALORIES:	
TIME (minutes):	

EXERCISES	SETS	Duration	Intensity	Cal/Burn

Blood Sugar Log	Before	After	Insulin
Breakfast			
Lunch			
Dinner			
Bedtime			

Note

Mood

My Results

Body Measurements/Sizing

Weight (pounds)	
Waist (inches)	
Chest (inches)	
Hips (inches)	
Estimated Lean Body Weight	
Body Fat Weight Estimated	
Body Fat Percentage Estimated Body Mass Index (BMI)	

Total Weight Lost ____________________

www.ingramcontent.com/pod-product-compliance
Lightning Source LLC
Chambersburg PA
CBHW082335270726
48658CB00017B/2856